CLEOPATRA ACI
IS NO MYT..

How to Cure your Acne and Get the Beauty of a Supermodel in Amazing step by step scientific proven diet and skin program
(For Teens)

M. KOTB M.D.

WHY I WROTE THIS BOOK

I wrote this book because of sarah. Let us listen to her

Sarah says: pimples Took Over My whole World

My face used to be so painful. I had oozing sores and rough darkish scabs on my chin and my mouth that I couldn't cover.

And i had severe compulsion to pick at them, i might decide pick at them at work, within the lavatory , feeling utter disgrace and disgust and even more so when my co-staff couldn't conceal their horror.

Going to work some days was once a nightmare and that i undoubtedly called in sick if matters were specially bad.

I would see eyes glancing around my face at my zits instead of looking me in the eyes.

I'd spend hours getting ready to see friends and popping my zits and applying make-up.

I would most likely be hours late when you consider the stress I had over my appearance.

And plenty of the time i'd simply cancel all collectively.

I simply felt so ashamed. I had random strangers comment to me about my skin . I had neighbors say, oh, they simply thought that I always had acne and that's just the way I used to be Discovering Cleopatra acne bath

That's once I did a google search, skin picking and zits. The book of dr kotb "Cleopatra acne bath is not a myth" came up.

I realized first about hormones and how they operate.

Dr kotb stated that a variety of persons think we can't change hormones, but we can!

Nearly all of my adult acne was cystic jawline zits (which i tried to pop earlier).

I also discovered about powerful herbs, otc, laser and much more .

My skin got much better untill it is one hundred%.

After allmy my life changed I found myself within the pleasant relationship i've ever been in, with the love of my life.

I confessed to him about how zits controlled my life and i established everything I did daily on it and the way it affected all of my choices.

He wiped away my tears and sent a thanks letter to the individual who helped me most, Dr. Kotb "

WHY YOU SHOULD READ THIS BOOK

What if there were secrets to cure your acne without having to go on some crazy diet.... just by doing these simple things?

And do all that with one affordable products that doesn't break the bank!

Not knowing what I'm going to teach you in this book kept me in the same old loop... struggling with acne nd pimples that just wouldn't budge... seeing my face gets pigmentations for absolutely no reason, regardless of how good my diet was... having to use sticky-notes to remember almost everything!

Learning to use these secrets was a game changer for me and it can be for you, too.

I've been involved in natural and medical healing for over 30 years, in my personal life, as a researcher and a practitioner. I know how long it takes to find reliable information and then figure out how to use it effectively. I've done that for you here.

In this book you are going to learn:

Top Five Things to Know About Acne

Can Your Diet Really Affect Your Acne?

Is There a real Link Between your Food and your Acne?

Does Drinking Milk Cause Acne?

Does Touching Your Face Cause Acne?

Does Masturbation Cause your Acne in Males?

4 Things You Should Never Do When Caring for Your Acne-Prone Skin

Do you know What Is the Difference Between a Pimple and a Blackhead?

6 Simple Ways To Prevent Adult Acne

8 Ways You May Be Making Your Acne Worse

7 Tiny Natural Changes That will Heal your Acne

Top 10 Home Remedies for Acne you can try today

will Rubbing Alcohol Clear your Acne?

Does Turmeric Clear Acne and Acne Scars?

Does Olive Oil Heal Acne Scars?

Will Coconut Oil Clear your Acne or Acne Marks?

Does Aloe Vera Clear Acne and Scars?

Will a Cinnamon Mask Clear your Acne or Acne Scars?

will Honey Clear your Acne?

Is an Egg Mask Good for your Acne?

Will Going Vegan Clear your Acne?

will Apple Cider Vinegar Clear your Acne?

will Tea Tree Oil Treat your Acne?

Does Using Toothpaste on your Pimples Really Work?

Can Urine Clear your Acne? Should You Put Pee

on your Pimples?

Top 4 Essential Oils for Acne

The Worst Acne Home Remedies you didn't know

Is it OK to Wear Makeup with Acne?

 6 Things You Can Do to Prevent Your Makeup from Causing
Pimples

5 Acne Treatment Myths Debunked

4 Important Acne Skin Care Steps

What Works, What Doesn't , and How To Use Them to Heal Your
Pimples

Acne Treatment Tips in Skin of Color

How To Choose an Effective OTC Acne Treatment Product for
Your Acne .

create 4 steps - At-Home OTC acne treatment regimen That
Works for You

4 Steps to Help You Get the Perfect Cleanser for Your Acne-Prone
Skin

5 Inexpensive Benzoyl Peroxide Cleansers for Treating your Acne at Home

Will you need to Treat your Acne with Topical Erythromycin

Will you need to Treat your Acne with Oral Erythromycin

Answers to the Most 6 Common Questions About Cleansing Your Acne-Prone Skin:

Are bar soaps OK?

Should I use a washcloth or scrubbing pads?

What temperature water should I use?

How often should I cleanse my face?

Do Pore Strips Work?

Is It Ever OK to Pop a Pimple or Squeeze a Blackhead?

Before you go to Popping, Try These Tricks

6 ways To Heal a Pimple That You've Picked, Popped or Squeezed

How to heal your Acne FAST before Your Wedding Day : Acne Treatment Tips for the Bride and Groom

How To Shave The Right Way When You Have Acne

Why OTC Acne Products Don't Work: 3 Fast Fixes for Getting Results from Over-the-Counter Acne Products

Why Pimples Come Back When You Stop Using Acne Medicine

Post-Inflammatory Hyperpigmentation : Is it a True Acne Scar?

Cortisone Shots for Acne is it good for you ?

Should you use Acne laser Surgery ? and How They will Help your Skin ?

Should You See an Esthetician Or Dermatologist For Acne ?

How to Care for buttocks Acne ?

Teen Acne

10 Things You Must Know About Treating Teen Acne in Boys

10 Things Teen Girls Should Know About Acne

Simple Tips for Treating Teen Acne

Acne Treatment for College Students

Acne Got You Down? : 5 Ways to Keep Depression away and Feel More Confident

Follow the advice in this book and you can start saving your skin and improving your health.

Carol, a housewife from Arizona says: "I'm speechless. It all makes sense now.. I can't believe I've never heard of this before."

"Your book saved my life. A million times thank you because you helped me avoid going crazy." -- amber from Houston, TX

Don't stay stuck in that rut, just wishing and getting nowhere. Be the person you want to be and have the health you want to live.

What's stopping you from achieving the health and body you deserve?

TABLE OF CONTENTS

WHY I WROTE THIS BOOK

WHY YOU SHOULD READ THIS BOOK

Cleopatra acne bath is no myth

The top 5 Tips you must know about Acne

Can Your Diet Really Affect Your Acne?

    Carbohydrates

    Chocolate and acne .

    Fried foods and Acne

    Milk and Dairy products

    Organic Diet

    Sugar

    Vegetarian and Vegan Diets

    Does ingesting Milk rationale pimples?

    Does Milk trigger acne ?

    The No-Dairy Philosophy

    Does Touching Your Face motive acne?

    Does Masturbation rationale acne in adult males?

    Don't ignore acne -- it can be treated!

Easy methods to deal with moderate acne

    6 easy methods To hinder adult acne

8 approaches you can be Making Your pimples Worse

7 Tiny common changes That Healed My acne

prime 10 home remedies for pimples that you could try today

top 10 home remedies for acne to check out today

dwelling cures for acne   Scars

ultimate hints for acne

Normal acne remedies That Work

Does Turmeric Clear acne and pimples Scars?

Does Olive Oil Heal acne   Scars?

   For Pitted Scars, do that

   Will Coconut Oil Clear pimples or acne Marks?

   Does Aloe Vera Clear acne   and Scars?

   will Honey Clear your acne?

   Is an Egg mask good in your acne ?

   Will Going Vegan Clear your pimples?

   Will Apple Cider Vinegar Clear your acne ?

   Will Tea Tree Oil treat your acne?

   Can Urine Clear your pimples? Will have to you set Pee on your pimples?

Top 4 principal Oils for acne

The Worst acne   home therapies you didn't know

OTC treatments

4 major pimples skin Care Steps

Acne treatment pointers in skin of colour

Treating acne with Topical Erythromycin

   Treating acne with Oral Erythromycin

6 approaches To Heal a Pimple that you've Picked, Popped or Squeezed

acne   remedy hints for the Bride and Groom

The right way to Shave The right means you probably have pimples

Why OTC acne   products do not Work:

Post-Inflammatory Hyperpigmentation : Is it a real pimples Scar?

Over-the-Counter remedies

Will have to You See an Esthetician Or Dermatologist For acne

Methods to handle buttocks pimples ?

10 things You have to learn about Treating Teen pimples in Boys

10 matters Teen girls should learn about acne

　　Use the proper makeup.

Top smart ways to treat acne   for tuition students

Dead Sea Mud Face Masks at Home: How to Use Dead Sea Mud Masks

　　Ingredients Used In Dead Sea Mud Masks:

Beauty secrets OF CLEOPATRA

Cleopatra acne bath is no myth

The beauty of Queen Cleopatra fascinated many ladies for thousands of years.

She is without doubt one of the most noted figures of vintage times and her repute stays alive uptill now.

What was her secret?

Why her character is surrounded by legends?

What are the sweetness secrets of Cleopatra?

Surely, Cleopatra was very exceptional lady and she adored herself, but she also knew how to use beauty secrets of her time.

We'll speak about some magnificence recommendations that Queen Cleopatra took advantage of ,peculiarly her no myth acne bath ,however her first beauty tip was her Invisible ingredient of magnificence.

Cleopatra knew that physical magnificence can appeal to the attention (that is why she took such an excellent care of her skin and physique),

intellect will make her the fascinating and skillful communicator (this is the reason Cleopatra loved to read books, study new matters and grow mentally), however she additionally knew about one invisible, but important ingredient of female magnificence – charm ;

 she knew that, if you wish to be irresistible and real attractive, it's fundamental to cultivate the inner confidence and inside attraction of a real woman!

try attempting one of the magnificence secrets for yourself and you are going to feel and seem as beautiful, as the beauty queen!

However to understand the beauty secrets of cleopatra

let us begin with the top 5 Tips you must know about Acne

The top 5 Tips you must know about Acne

although we do not know the whole thing there's to find out about why some men and women get acne whilst others do not, there are plenty of matters we do know about how it develops and what will also can be done about it.

1. Pimples are induced by means of three ESSENCIAL causes.

There are many myths about what explains zits.

So just know that because you've eaten chocolate or touched your face, you haven't done anything to motive your zits.

In fact, there's no specific reason of acne.

Rather, it's an effect of many reasons coming together:

we know that people with zits are likely to have overactive sebaceous glands—the glands that make our skin 's oil.

Acne-susceptible skin also does not shed useless dead cells as readily. It also has a bigger amount of Propionibacteria acnes—micro organism linked to inflamed acne blemishes—within the pores.different factors that make contributions to zits progress include oily cosmetics, comedogenic skin care or hair care products, precise drugs such as steroids, and estrogen medicinal drugs.pimples also tends to run in families. If your father and mother had zits at any point of their lives, your risk of developing it is bigger.

2. All breakouts begin as a blocked pore.

All acne blemishes form when oil and dead skin cells become trapped within the hair follicle, creating a plug inside the pore. This plug of lifeless cells and oil is referred to as a comedo (plural for comedo is comedones).

Blackheads and whiteheads are examples of non-inflamed comedones.

Because the breakout progresses and bacteria invade, the wall of the hair follicle can rupture inside the skin , developing infection and redness.

Inflamed blemishes range in severity depending on the injury to the follicle wall and the quantity of infection present.

Severe injury to the follicle can create deeper lesions and cysts.

1-Hormones set off pimples progress. There may be a purpose why acne most of the time develops during puberty—all those hormones are raging.

During puberty, there is a surge of androgen hormones inside the body.

Androgen hormones, certainly testosterone, greatly impact acne progress.

Additionally they stimulate the sebaceous glands, developing an oilier complexion and another prone to breakouts.

Moreover to puberty, females may even see tremendous hormonal fluctuations in the course of menstruation, being pregnant, menopause, and perimenopause.

For the period of these lifestyles phases, acne is definitely to develop or flare up.

1-Zits can happen at (virtually) any age.

We consider of acne as being a teenage difficulty, but that's now not the case in any respect.

Of course, teen acne and preteen zits is common.

But pimples is just not constrained to young adults.

Many guys and females have adult-onset acne breakouts.

Zits may also arise in infants, little toddlers, and children.

Truly, if in case you have skin , you can get pimples!

3. There are a lot of distinct varieties of pimples. Do you know there are lots of forms of zits?

Zits vulgaris is the technical time period in your average acne breakouts and it is essentially the most usual type of zits.

It could possibly differ in severity. With moderate acne vulgaris, you can have simply minor blemishes.

More inflamed, widespread breakouts are considered moderate acne.

Srvere acne vulgaris can be broken down even further depending on the type of blemishes present on the skin.

Nodular pimples is a severe form of acne vulgaris.

Men and women with nodular pimples have deep, infected breakouts referred to as nodules. Nodules have an effect on deeper layers of the skin than typical pimples.

Cystic zits is a further extreme variety of zits that causes painful cysts.

Zits cysts are different than pimples. Cysts are deep, fluid-stuffed blemishes that quite often have to be drained by a dermatologist.

Nodular pimples is a term used to describe severe pimples vulgaris that causes both nodules and zits cysts.

Comedonal zits is a type of non-inflammatory pimples. Instead of inflamed zits, men and women with get blackheads, milia and closed comedones. The skin looks and feels hard and bumpy.

Got zits on your back and shoulders the place your backpack rests?

Or to your forehead underneath your hat band? You have zits mechanica. This kind of pimples develops the place there may be extra warmth, pressure, or friction on the dead .

 It's very common for athletes to increase this sort of acne where garb or sporting activities apparatuses rests or rubs.

Pimples cosmetica is a type of zits that is precipitated by using hair care or cosmetic merchandise clogging the pores.

Suspect this form of acne in the event you've begun breaking out after commencing a new beauty product or if you are breaking out in a certain situation (like round your hairline where you follow pomades or hairspray).

Excoriated pimples isn't brought about with the aid of the causes that set off zits vulgaris.

Rather, excoriated acne is created by picking at blemishes

Occasionally popping acne doesn't motive excoriated pimples. It develops when the picking out becomes compulsive and damages the skin .

acne rosacea is a skin situation that also causes redness and acne. Unlike zits vulgaris, rosacea appears only throughout the face (above all the cheeks, nostril, and chin) and not on the body.

Although we do not know exactly what causes rosacea, doctors speculate it is usually the result of a bacterium, microscopic mite, or readily sensitive capillaries.

Can Your Diet Really Affect Your Acne?

Is There a real link Between your meals and your acne ?

There is so much knowledge out there about food and acne.

Some professionals declare certain foods can cause pimples, and slicing these meals from your diet program can improve acne .

Others say there's no link between food and acne so that diet plan has nothing to do with the health of your skin.

The place does the truth lay? In general somewhere in the middle.

Let's attempt to find it out.

Carbohydrates

not all carbs are equal and, in accordance to some stories, the flawed types could affect your skin .

Researchers have determined that high glycemic index meals (think white bread, potatoes, and sugary junk foods) appear to make acne worse.

A diet program rich in low glycemic index foods, which involves wheat bread, wheat pasta, legumes and different whole grains, seems to improve pimples in young adults.

Much more research wants to be accomplished to prove, somehow, that carbohydrates have any result on pimples.

Nonetheless, you particularly don't have anything to lose by means of altering to a more healthy food plan.

This sweet has been blamed for many a case of acne.

How many of us were warned to keep away from chocolate if we wish clear skin?

Good information for all you chocoholics in the market: Chocolate does not cause pimples.

Correctly, more knowledge is coming out displaying that chocolate (the darker the easier) is without a doubt excellent for you.

Dark chocolate is filled with healthful antioxidants.

Does eating oily foods translate to oily skin?

Chalk this one up as one more pimples-explanations myth.

There isn't any way to hide French fries, fried bird, and other deep-fried morsels as wellbeing food, but they don't make your skin extra oily. They won't make acne worse either.

Milk and Dairy products

A number of reviews have proven a link between pimples severity and consumption of milk and different dairy products.

It is still a stretch to assert that milk causes acne, and giving up all dairy in general won't reason acne to disappear.

Nonetheless, should you're a significant milk drinker, you may need to scale back on the dairy for a while and see if it has any influence on your skin .

those healthy grapes, tomatoes, and apples are amazingly tasty.

And it is fun to browse the farmer's marketplace for new and detailed natural and organic fare.

However will loading your diet with natural meals help to clear your skin ?

Whilst there are various distinctive causes to go organic, clearing up pimples is not one among them.

No matter what some natural proponents say, the research simply would not back this up.

Consuming natural foods may just curb the amount of pesticides you take in, however there is not any indication that it has any result on acne   breakouts.

So, if the price of organic food gives you sticker shock, forgoing it for regular produce won't hurt your skin.

at the same time some individuals swear consuming sugary foods makes their acne worse, the research linking sugar to pimples development is weak.

A handful of small reviews endorse there is a link but the pool of contributors used to be particularly small.

Also, they relied on individuals self-reporting pimples breakouts— not an objective way to categorise alterations within the skin.

From the understanding we have right now, it appears sugar doesn't play any role in acne progress.

interestingly, a diet rich in meat may elevate your probabilities of constructing acne via a problematic chain response.

There is a protein-complex within the human physique that some researchers feel is responsible for turning on this chain response that stimulates the skin 's oil glands and makes acne breakouts more likely to advance.

The trigger to get this process started is the amino acid leucine.

Foods like beef and chicken are naturally high in leucine.

So far, there isn't any definitive proof, as that is only a concept.

But it is an interesting look at how the skin works.

We do understand, although, that pimples development is very complicated and it can be extremely not going that just altering one aspect of your diet goes to thoroughly resolve a case of acne .

Does ingesting Milk rationale pimples?

Some doctors consider that what we eat could certainly have an effect on our skin and make acne worse. Exceedingly, they're no longer pointing fingers at chocolate or potato chips, however rather at milk.

That's correct -- the healthful drink that we have always regarded healthy is getting a contemporary look.

Some research has shown a correlation between milk consumption and the incidence of acne. It seems milk drinkers increase extra extreme acne than non-milk drinkers.

One learn, published in the may 2008 challenge of the Journal of the American Academy of Dermatology, seemed at the diets of teenaged boys. The younger men who drank probably the most milk additionally tended to have the worst pimples.

This helps the outcome of prior reports, during which teenage ladies had been requested to keep meals diaries and reveal breakout endeavor. Again, ladies whose diets were wealthy in dairy products had extra extreme pimples than the leisure.

Of all dairy products, milk used to be the worst culprit. Chocolate milk, cottage cheese, and sherbet also had a bad outcomes on the dead . However different dairy products didn't look to intent breakouts.

Apparently, skim milk brought about breakouts extra quite often than whole milk, so it appears fat content in milk is not the wrongdoer. And those who took diet D supplements did not have more breakouts, so nutrition D isn't concept to be the purpose either.

Fatty foods additionally didn't trigger breakouts.

And the foods that many people accomplice with inflicting acne --
chocolate, pizza, soda and French fries -- didn't look to increase
breakout activity at all.

How would Milk have an effect on the dead ?

Why would certain dairy merchandise make contributions to acne
? Some believe it can be the hormones found in milk. Milk
involves androgen hormones, which have long been related to the
formation of acne breakouts.

Testosterone is an androgen hormone, and it is strongly linked to
acne development. It can be most traditionally proposal of as a
male hormone, however women produce testosterone too, despite
the fact that in lesser quantities.

Testosterone, by way of a elaborate chain reaction, creates
dihydrotestosterone (DHT). DHT stimulates the sebaceous glands,
developing an oilier skin that's extra prone to pore blockages and,
eventually, acne.

Milk naturally is full of hormones, together with DHT. It is viable
that milk comprises ample hormones to affect the physique,
including the skin . Men and women who're genetically
predisposed to pimples breakouts will have a much better reaction
to the hormones in milk, in accordance to some researchers.

The IGF-1 progress aspect

Many dairy farmers also provide their cows further hormones to stimulate milk creation and enable the cow to provide more milk. Therefore, most milk may be very high in IGF-1.

IGF-1 is a growth aspect that peaks in the human body for the duration of youth when acne is generally at it is worst.

It is believed that IGF-1, together with testosterone and DHT, set off acne breakouts.

In several experiences, high milk consumption was linked to excessive IGF-1 phases. Once more, skim milk was once related to greater IGF-1 levels than entire milk.

The processing of skim milk may give an explanation for why it's linked to pimples severity extra normally than whole milk. Whey proteins are added to offer skim milk a creamier consistency. Some speculate that these proteins influence pimples progress.

A hyperlink Between Dairy products and pimples Severity

That means that drinking a glass of milk, even a number of glasses of milk every day, isn't going to purpose anyone with otherwise clear skin to suddenly breaking out in acne.

It is principal to have an understanding of that none of the reviews have shown proof constructive that milk reasons pimples. Actually, they exhibit simplest a viable hyperlink between dairy merchandise and pimples severity.

That signifies that drinking a glass of milk, even a couple of glasses of milk every day, is not going to reason anyone with or else clear skin to abruptly start breaking out in acne. The research indicates that consuming milk may make acne worse for humans who're already breakout-prone.

Disagreement amongst scientific gurus

Of direction, not every body who drinks a number of milk breaks out in pimples, and many disagree with these findings. The Dairy Council counters that the outcome are skewed, citing the truth that in a single study, adult ladies were requested about their dairy consumption during the years after they left excessive tuition.

And plenty of clinical experts are wary of the conclusions being drawn, due to the fact that they do not don't forget other factors that will affect pimples severity. They're also quick to factor out that the reviews don't link milk to acne development; they simply establish a correlation between milk consumption and acne severity.

The biggest crisis for researchers is proving this idea. There's no solution to do a double-blind, randomized controlled trial (viewed the gold normal in research), in view that there may be nothing that can be utilized as an adequate placebo for milk.

There may be nonetheless no rough proof proving milk consumption reasons, and even worsens, acne . Far more study is needed earlier than this idea can be demonstrated.

nonetheless, some doctors are taking a new view of how weight-reduction plan impacts the dead , and this no-dairy philosophy has its believers. Some dermatologists say they've had success in having their patients cut milk and dairy from their diets.

Is milk a set off for you? Most effective which you could tell. If you are a giant milk drinker, you would need to cut it out of your weight loss plan for a number of months to peer for those who detect an growth for your skin , specially in case your acne is not responding good to more conventional cures.

Don't forget, acne tends to wax and wane all on its own, too. So, to particularly test out this theory for your self, you'll ought to reduce dairy from your weight loss plan for several months to get a excellent consider if it can be working for you.

Acne medication

even if banning milk from your eating regimen appears to make stronger your acne , it obviously won't be ample to totally clear your skin . For that, you can want an acne healing medication.

Over-the-counter products would work in case your acne is slight. However most men and women get the high-quality outcome from prescription acne medicines.

You will have perpetually touched your face with your palms and in no way given it a second suggestion. That's, except your pal told you that touching your face with your fingers explanations acne, and if you happen to stopped doing it, your acne would leave.

Might it fairly be that easy to clear your skin ?

With ease touching your face isn't causing your acne.

The whole suggestion that touching your face together with your fingers explanations acne has been overstated.

Touching your face along with your hands, at the same time now not particularly important, most commonly is not doing a lot to intent acne . And, extra importantly, with no trouble no longer touching your face anymore is not going to make acne go away.

Acne is brought about by way of several causes ; fingers should not one in every of them.

The rationale you have acne is just not considering the fact that you brushed your fingers throughout your cheek last week, and it can be no longer even seeing that you wish to leisure your chin for your hand.

The true acne -inflicting culprits are: over-lively sebaceous glands (sometimes called oil glands), irregular shedding of skin cells, targeted bacteria (certainly propionibacterium acnes), and hormonal influences. Touching, or not touching, the skin is not going to influence these causes all that so much, if in any respect.

Squeezing or picking out at acne   is under no circumstances a just right notion.

Of direction, this all depends on what form of touching we're speaking about. There are matters your palms can do on the way to make acne   worse.

Settling on at the dead , squeezing blemishes, and scratching off scabs will undoubtedly make acne seem worse. While you pop a pimple or pick at a blemish scab, you're creating more irritation and detrimental your skin .

So, in this case, a hands-off procedure is certainly the pleasant wager. However determining at the skin may be very special than merely touching your face.

Touching your face is not always invaluable, though.

This isn't to claim you you're now free to touching and rubbing at the skin with abandon. Your fingers are not normally the cleanest things within the entire world, so you may also no longer want to be touching your face a ton anyway.

It is also a excellent concept to clean your palms earlier than touching your face, even if it's to not scale down pimples. Hands can harbor germs. Touching your mouth, nose, or eyes with dirty hands can unfold matters like cold and flu viruses.

And if you are a bona-fide picker, it as a rule is pleasant for you now not touch your face at all. If you feel a pimple, it is tough to battle the urge to decide upon at it, is not it? On this case, it's so a lot simpler to prevent temptation altogether with the aid of now not touching the face within the first place.

Different things touching your face can set off a breakout.

Although touching your face together with your fingers isn't a gigantic acne-inflicting trigger, some matters touching your face can actually make pimples worse. These are items like sweat bands, hats, soccer helmets etc.

It is more concerning the friction, though, than spreading micro organism. Acne that's prompted by way of friction is known as acne mechanica.

So, you could not need to spend a lot of time together with your face resting to your palms for simply that motive, too. In the event you do that rather a lot (like everyday during a boring class interval) you may observe an increase in breakouts in that discipline.

Again, that is more from consistent stress on the skin , no longer from a mere touch. And, for lots of humans, even plenty of resting cheeks on hands would not have an impact on pimples a method or one more.

Not touching your face will not resolve pimples, but a good cure product will.

However even supposing you were to by no means, ever touch your face from this factor on, you'll nonetheless have pimples. Because acne isn't induced by without difficulty touching your face, pimples can not be "cured" through not touching your face. Not touching your face will not stop acne.

If you want to see actual development on your skin, you ought to get on an acne medication routine. This can be over-the-counter products, but it might imply prescription medications too. A excellent daily skin care movements, a verified acne medicine, consistent therapy and a little of time will do the most to banish these breakouts, regardless of whether you are touching your face or not.

Yes, I'm going there.

So, the topic of masturbation causing acne   is anything that i have located comes up as a rule around the web – commonly in the type of stories that say 'no, there's absolutely no correlation' juxtoposed against guys who swear up and down that masturbating causes them to interrupt out.

Women, i'll say right now – i have not ever heard/learn of any females finding that masturbation reasons pimples, so that you can breathe effortless as this does look to be often a male difficulty.

So… anyway, back to the question, does masturbation cause acne in adult males?

Good, to be sincere, i'd say no – masturbation does no longer "purpose" pimples. Pimples is a manifestation of underlying problems – gut problems and dietary deficiencies, if you want my opinion. Which i guess you do if you happen to're reading my internet site. However, once you've got that happening (and most do to a few degree), persons look to have a few bajillion specific things that may set off their acne.

For instance, one individual's primary set off may be stress, for others, it's a specified meals. Or probably it's fluoride within the water provide, blood sugar swings, or your chemical cleaner that's stressful the heck out of your skin .

Sadly for some guys in the market, intercourse and masturbation can also be one in every of them. This may not be true for each male, but judging via real men and women's experiences and no longer the stories (I opt for actual humans's experiences), there could also be a link right here.

For illustration, I obtained this e mail from someone the previous day:

hi Tracy!

I've been staring at your videos, and i attempted them out, and any other stuff as well. And i discovered something... strange.

Consider me, I'm not trolling, this isn't a comic story. I'm a 20 years historic male, and i found out that masturbation CAN rationale very extreme acne .

I was on paleo weight loss plan, threw away the cosmetics, etc.

Good, my face obtained beautiful just right, but after I masturbate, it will get fairly bad, like 30 acne out of nowhere. Good, I couldn't understand it earlier than, considering the fact that I ate junk food and stuff, but now, when all unhealthy factors where eradicated, i've noticed it. My skin Got particularly bad on sunday, and i said to myself: i cannot masturbate, but consume the same meals as before.

My skin is lovely powerful now in comparison with the old days, and that i handiest needed to stop that ONE thing: masturbation. Not given that of junk meals, or some other thing.

Long story short: masturbation might be a significant element (its as a minimum 80% for me, the other 19 is settling on the pimples, and 1 is the food) probably considering the fact that it tilts the hormone stability?

Now, it appears to me like it is a bit of an severe case – and that i've constantly been hesitant to mention this knowledge set off when you consider that I didn't need any individual to get all paranoid about this natural act if it wasn't the offender.

However I figured it used to be time to speak about it due to the fact the evidence is particularly clear to me that there's knowledge for acne production right here, accordingly, you guys out there might want to try experimenting with cutting yourself off for a while to peer what occurs.

Why Would Masturbation trigger acne ?

That I don't be aware of for certain, but the customary idea is that the surge of testosterone while you grow to be aroused triggers it. Male androgens, finally, are liable for end reactions in the acne formation cycle.

This idea is sensible to me considering that i've additionally heard that in some men, heavy weight lifting exercises that broaden testosterone construction may also set off pimples.

Nonetheless, another conception that I to find exciting is that it's no longer the hormone surge, however the vitamins and minerals lost when you ejaculate. It appears semen contains vitamins B6, B12, and E; Calcium; Magnesium; Selenium; and Zinc.

Zinc in unique is a mineral that is relatively principal to healthy skin and its deficiency has a powerful hyperlink to acne. So i can see how this conception would make feel, exceptionally on the grounds that i've heard that, more often than not (now not acne related), that many men to find that they have extra total power once they hold again.

However (no pun intended), it also doesn't make experience to me, on the grounds that your physique is constantly making use of these vitamins and minerals to create the sperm and semen within your body whether or not you blow your load or not. Despite the fact that maybe production goes into overdrive afterwards to be able to trap up, and in case you are masturbating everyday or more than one times a day, you then relatively are draining yourself of life drive and central vitamins and minerals.

In short, I don't comprehend the truth and considering there are not any reviews confirming whatever, we handiest have speculation.

I ought to decide on Between sex and acne ? Nice. Kill Me Now.

Good, notably if the "ejaculation loses vitamins and minerals" thought is proper, it doesn't mean that you simply ought to absolutely give up – simply minimize a little. Try to do it twice a week simplest, well spaced out. But of course, you'll need to test to look what works for you, as every person is exceptional.

I entirely realise that looking to opt for between pimples and orgasms isn't a enjoyable thing to do. So I asked the person who sent me the above email how he felt about this. I stated:

i've a question – and that is – are you planning to certainly not masturbate or have sex EVER once more? It's a lovely tough factor to decide on between. I've heard it's extra to do with ejaculation and the vitamins and minerals (peculiarly zinc) that a male loses, so as a result, it wouldn't be too detrimental for those who just did it a couple of times every week spread out as an alternative of certainly not.

Anyway, I just wanted to understand how you're resolving that a part of it with yourself…. You need to be completely satisfied that you would be able to control your acne, but it surely's at rather the rate. Or is giving it up not the sort of large deal to you?

And he mentioned:

Im simply gonna curb it to as soon as per week for now, and see the outcome. Naturally i'll do them, but more sparingly. You'll't stop doing these, considering the fact that without them life wouldn't be full. Acne is unhealthy, but lifestyles without intercourse is worse.

And there you've it.

Four things You will have to not ever Do When Caring in your acne

 excellent dead SKIN care is a principal a part of your acne healing routine. What to do to maintain your skin , however do you know what you will have to not do? Don't sabotage your healing hobbies via making these acne dead   care errors.

Do not pop pimples.

Certain, you can be ready to extract some gunk from a pimple, however a whole lot extra is going down below the dead 's surface.

When a pimple is squeezed, the follicle wall is put under extreme strain. If the wall bursts, contaminated fabric spills from the pore and into the skin .

Even supposing you get some pus out of the pimple, extra damage is being achieved to the dead . That is why the pimple mostly finally ends up looking worse, redder and infected after you've popped it.

Worse, you also run the threat of scarring. So don't pop, squeeze, or otherwise prefer at your blemishes.

Don't scrub your breakouts.

It appears we're all tempted to clean at our breakouts. However blemishes can't be scrubbed away. Scrubbing would not avert acne from forming either.

Correctly, too much scrubbing can motive irritation, redness, and infection. In short, scrubbing can make your pimples seem and believe a entire lot worse.

Remember, your skin is a sensitive organ and will have to be treated gently. This means no ultra-gritty scrubs, abrasive cleaning pads, or fiercely rubbing at your skin with a washcloth.

As an alternative, wash your skin with moderate cleaning soap or cleanser making use of simply your fingers or a soft cloth. These electrical facial cleaning brushes are adequate, provided the bristles are delicate they usually don't irritate your skin .

Do not use too many therapy merchandise directly, or follow them too probably.

Although it's tempting, slathering on topical medications on numerous times day-to-day will not clear acne faster. However it will go away your skin super dry and annoyed.

Use a couple of acne cures directly (for instance, salicylic acid lotion, on prime of benzoyl peroxide cream, on top of Retin A gel) and you'll be able to additionally run the threat of over-drying and irritating your skin.

Don't layer merchandise to your skin. Alternatively, area applications throughout the day -- like making use of your salicylic acid purifier in the morning, benzoyl peroxide lotion at night. In the event you discover any infection, lower use to each different day or drop the second product altogether.

In case you are making use of prescription acne medications, in no way use a different acne product with out first getting your health care provider's adequate. Specified acne medications just isn't used collectively. For example, benzoyl peroxide will inactivate Retin-A (tretinoin) when applied together. And when you apply it to prime of Aczone (dapsone) it may possibly flip your skin orange (albeit quickly).

Don't ignore acne -- it can be treated!

Pimples can be cleared, and there are therapy options that can help.

If pimples is mild, you've gotten only a few random pimples and blackheads, you can first are attempting an over-the-counter remedy.

However should you are attempting OTC acne cures for a number of weeks and you're now not seeing outcome, make an appointment together with your physician. Your dermatologist has a lot of prescription drugs just for clearing pimples.

So don't wait to see if acne will go away on its own. You can be surprised on the therapy choices available. So, put in a call to your dermatologist. The earlier you start cure, the sooner you'll see development.

Have you learnt what is the change Between a Pimple and a Blackhead?

What is the difference between a blackhead and a pimple? Each acne and blackheads are varieties of acne blemishes. But each one appears another way for your skin, and each and every is dealt with in a different way too.

Acne are inflamed.

pimples are a variety of inflamed blemish. Pimple are pink and swollen. They mostly harm, but not perpetually.

Some acne stay small, but others can get quite gigantic. Pimples can show up on the face, neck, shoulders and upper torso subject.

Blackheads aren't inflamed.

Blackheads are a kind of non-infected blemish. They are often flat, they are not purple or swollen, and they don't harm. In fact, you would no longer even become aware of you have a blackhead until you're rather inspecting your skin within the mirror.

That you may get blackheads within the identical locations pimples appear, however they may be most long-established on the nose, chin, around the lips, and in the ears.

Acne have a purple or white head.

There are honestly unique varieties of acne (crazy, right?) A pimple with a crimson head, or only a crimson bump on the skin , is known as a papule.

Your pimple may advance a white or yellow pus-filled top. If it does, it's now known as a pustule. Now not all papules change into pustules, though.

Pustules are often called "whiteheads." simply to make things more intriguing (or confusing) there's a further sort of blemish that's also known as a whitehead -- milia.

Even though they share the identical nickname, milia and acne are fully exceptional varieties of blemishes.

Blackheads have a depressing brown or black head.

Blackheads have a depressing black head, for that reason the identify. The appear like a gloomy dot on the skin . Have a "freckle" show up that has under no circumstances been there before? Appear intently -- it can be usually a blackhead.

Some blackheads are super tiny, so small that you could barely see them. Other blackheads can get rather gigantic, several millimeters in diameter.

The technical title for a blackhead is open comedo.

Pimples advance when oil and useless skin cells turn out to be trapped in the pore.

acne   boost when a plug of oil and lifeless dead   cells becomes trapped shrink in the follicle.

Oil is still pumped into the plugged follicle, with nowhere to go. Add in some typical skin micro organism, p. Acnes, and the follicle becomes irritated and engorged. The follicle wall breaks, white blood cells rush in, and the pore turns into red and swollen. Voila! A pimple has shaped.

Blackheads improve when a blockage happens at the skin 's floor.

just like a pimple, blackheads additionally show up when a plug develops within the follicle.

Although it is going to appear like dust has end up trapped for your pore, that black spot isn't dust in any respect. It's truly a plug of your skin 's oil that has end up trapped on the dead 's floor. The top of the plug oxidizes and turns into that dark blackish-brown spot your see.

Here's how you can treat pimples.

There are plenty of pimple-busting products and medications to be had.

For minor breakouts, over-the-counter acne   medicinal drugs must do the trick.

More stubborn or widespread acne   will also be dealt with with prescription pimples medications that you just get from your health care professional.

Recall, don't pop inflamed acne!

Easy methods to deal with moderate acne

that is how you deal with blackheads.

Not like acne , that you could gently squeeze blackheads to cast off them (gently being the operative word).

Due to the fact you can extract blackheads your self, or have your esthetician extract them for you throughout a facial.

Pore strips are yet another approach to treat blackheads, despite the fact that the outcome are transitority.

If you wish to keep blackheads away for good, you need to get on a general cure application. Once more, moderate blackheads can also be handled with OTC products. Prescription medicinal drugs are nice for entrenched blackheads.

Ugh. You are a grown girl—maybe even battling satisfactory lines—and now...A pimple? Significantly? Adult pimples is increasingly long-established, but some handy steps can also be taken to nip these spots within the bud before they exhibit up for your face.

Devour the proper meals.

Greasy food doesn't cause a greasy face, however some meals could exacerbate an already-brewing condition. Simple carbs and sugar spike on your blood sugar and can trigger dead 's inflammatory response and provoke a breakout, says Linda k. Franks, MD, a dermatologist in NY city. In a similar fashion, several reviews have proven a hyperlink between dairy merchandise and pimples, probably since of the hormones which might be present in these foods. Buying healthy can support: typical dairy merchandise can come from hormone-fed animals, so they in general have extra hormones than their healthy counterparts.

And the unhealthy information? A small gain knowledge of provided on the February 2011 assembly of the Academy of Dermatology observed a correlation between the amount of chocolate that individuals consumed (only men have been studied, to be able to lessen the position of hormonal influence) and the number of pimples lesions they developed. (Get A Free Trial of Prevention + 12 Free gifts.)

hold your stress in determine as a lot as possible.

Stress raises the infection that leads to grownup acne breakouts, says Gil Yosipovitch, MD, a scientific professor of dermatology at Wake forest university. In the event you do have a stress-related breakout, soft your skin with a lotion containing dead -sloughing salicylic acid or micro organism-busting benzoyl peroxide, plus a noncomedogenic moisturizer so skin won't get too dry. (try this 5-minute manner that lowers your stress fifty five%.)

Use the proper basis.

To nix slick spots, are attempting an oil-free, long-lasting liquid (it stays matte longer) or a cream-to-powder formula; both contain silica, a powderlike ingredient that sops up shine. (verify out these foundations that take years off your appear.) If you're pimple-prone, use a base with acne-combating salicylic acid. Considering that oil and acne type mostly for your T-zone, use a groundwork brush to use; its tapered tip helps goal tough-to-attain nooks. Pro picks: Maybelline match Me Shine-Free groundwork ($9, maybelline.Com) or Almay Clear Complexion Blemish therapy makeup ($eight, ulta.Com).

Don't sleep together with your make-up on.

Please tell us you are now not doing this! Be sure to wash your face at night time with heat water or a gentle purifier (see subsequent tip).

Use a facial wash with salicylic acid.

"It will get into the pores and dislodges particles," says Diane Berson, MD, an assistant professor of dermatology at the Weill medical college of Cornell school and board member of the American pimples and Rosacea Society. Avert gel cleansers (they can incorporate alcohol) and granulated scrubs, which strip the skin of oil, making it overcompensate and produce more.

Use the vigour duo.

If salicylic acid doesn't work, try anything that mixes a retinoid with benzoyl peroxide. When researchers combined adapalene, a retinoid that reduces infection, with benzoyl peroxide, which kills the micro organism that reason acne , learn members' acne elevated on common by greater than 50% in 12 weeks—about 15% better than with both ingredient alone. "This combo healing ambitions three out of four reasons of acne," says Diane Thiboutot, MD, professor of dermatology at Penn State's Milton S. Hershey scientific core.

8 approaches you can be Making Your pimples Worse

you may feel you are doing everything which you could to deal with your pimples. However little matters could add up to make it worse. Do any of those errors sound familiar?

1. Your cellphone mobilephone Is soiled

think about it: Your face produces oil and sweat, which will get onto your mobilephone when you're on a name.

If you don't easy that off, for the duration of your next call you are pushing it back into your skin , along with any micro organism that has grown.

To scrub it, comply with the guidelines out of your telephone's maker. You might are trying ear buds or one other arms-free headset. Pressure from holding your mobile towards your cheek can also rationale breakouts by using annoying your skin .

2. You place Hair products Too just about Your Hairline

should you use an anti-frizz product, or a thick gel or pomade, observe it away from your forehead.

Otherwise, that you can get a line of pimples right there at your hair line.

3. You quit Too quickly

"every person wishes clear skin the day before today, however we have no silver bullet that works instantly; acne cures take weeks to start kicking in," says dermatologist Joshua Zeichner, MD, of Mt. Sinai health center in ny. He focuses on treating acne .

If over-the-counter acne merchandise don't support inside 2 to four weeks, then you may have to see a dermatologist. This is notably fundamental when you have acne cysts or in case your acne leaves scars.

4. You Wash Your Face too much

"one of the most greatest myths is: 'My face is soiled, and that is why i'm getting pimples,'" says dermatologist Whitney Bowe, MD, of evolved Dermatology P.C. In Westchester, N.Y.

"Washing too much can strip the skin of most important oils, main the body to satirically produce more oil, which can result in extra acne ," Zeichner says.

Washing twice a day is all you need.

5. You make mistakes when you Wash Your Face

do not use a soiled or damp washcloth while you wash. Micro organism can with no trouble construct up on them. Use a clean washcloth whenever.

Also, do not exfoliate too most commonly. Sandy or sugary products, tough scrubbing pads or loofahs, and even electric brushes can purpose tiny tears within the dead if used day-to-day. The effect is inflammation and infection.

That can make treating pimples trickier. Exfoliate handiest a few times a week, Zeichner says.

6. You employ an excessive amount of Zit Cream

"extra cream is just not necessarily better. Actually, [some] constituents can also be rather disturbing to the skin ," Zeichner says.

You may want less than you feel. "One inexperienced-pea-sized quantity is all you have to cover your face."

7. You decide on and dad acne

It's comprehensible to want to do away with acne   ASAP. However this distinct plan of attack can intent deeper issues.

"instead of clearing the blockage out, you are pushing it further down, and that may result in scarring," Zeichner says.

Alternatively, put a little treatment immediately onto the pimple to make it smaller and less infected.

Eight. You eat Too Many Sweets and Starchy foods

"When mom informed you to keep away from these objects, she could have been on to anything," Zeichner says.

No meals is established to cause pimples. But sugary, processed ones equivalent to white breads, white pasta, potato chips, cookies, and muffins may be linked to acne , says Bowe, who has researched this. There's no draw back to limiting sugary meals.

Some reports have linked dairy products to pimples, however that's not precise.

7 Tiny common changes That Healed My acne

no one likes acne . Blackheads are pests, whiteheads are embarrassing, and cystic irritation is exasperating. Worst of all, healing customarily includes harsh cleansers and prescription drugs. Fortunately, there are extra ordinary medication options on hand than ever before. I'm a massive fan of working with the totality of my body naturally to regulate a pattern, like pimples. I realized these 7 nontoxic tips from estheticians, dermatologists, and vigor healers alongside my three-12 months experience of treatment my acne. They'll take you simply 5 to 10 minutes a day, and would yield amazing sudden results like extra vigour, better digestion, and of path, much less acne.

(On just a quarter-acre of land, that you would be able to produce fresh, natural meals for a family of four—year-circular. Rodale's The outside homestead suggests you ways; get your replica at present.)

This tip is my favorite, considering i am a giant tea lover. It comes from my holistic dermatologist, Alan M. Dattner, MD, author of Radiant skin from the inside Out: The Holistic Dermatologist's advisor to healing Your skin Naturally. He recommends ingesting one cup of skin Detox tea by using Yogi every day. It has potent organic herbs in it like burdock, red clover, and honeybush leaf, which can be known liver detox, anti-inflammatory, and immune-strengthening herbs. It's caffeinated (however just 18 mg, compared with the ninety mg in eight ouncesof coffee), so every morning I repair myself a big cup with slightly of honey to kick-start my day.

Trade your pillowcase.

You spend about fifty six hours every week to your pillowcase—that is a lot of time to roll round in absorbed buildup from hair merchandise, make-up, and sweat, although you bathe at night time. "regardless of the material, pillowcases lure oil, grime, and micro organism," say dermatologists Lily Talakoub and Naissan Wesley. "change them day-to-day if viable." that is primarily fundamental you probably have a nightly face product movements to your pimples. You do not need it constructing up or getting to your hair even as you sleep. Besides, who does not love snuggling into a fresh pillow?

Consider this herb.

Lawn pest or acne   comfort? Additionally to sipping herbal tea, I've delivered dandelion root tincture to my routine. The phrase "dandelion" is taken from the Greek taraxos, which means sickness, and akos, which means remedy, in keeping with Rodale's Illustrated Encyclopedia of Herbs. "Dandelion root is a smooth liver herb that has a vaguely coffee-like style," says Dattner. Use it to help the liver, our body's giant filter, which separates vitamin from toxins and chemicals. If our liver isn't working correctly, the toxins are released into the bloodstream and might intent signs like pimples, explains Dattner. "Herbs are as a rule toward meals than medicinal drugs, so their margin of safeguard is higher," Dattner says, but he recommends consulting a legit before attempting a new herb, certainly if you are on another treatment.

Eat less dairy.

Consume less dairy.

If cheese is as colossal a staple for your weight-reduction plan as it used to be for me (responsible as charged), you may want to feel twice, on the grounds that it would exacerbate your acne . "Dairy merchandise have been proven to expand sebum production, which encourages the progress of acne," explains nutrition specialist Scott Schreiber, DCBCN, CNS, LDN. Sebum is the oily substance that maintains our hair and skin moisturized. When it is no longer in assess, it will possibly result in overly oily skin , and acne .

The hormone IGF-1 in milk has been linked to acne considering that it chronically stimulates your sebaceous glands. Try cutting dairy out for a month or two. When I did this, i spotted enormously less inflammation on my face. I substituted almond or coconut milk for the creamy stuff, and bought my recommended 1,000 mg of calcium a day from salmon, chinese cabbage, almonds, and oatmeal.

Restrict these hair merchandise.

preclude these hair merchandise.

Talakoub and Wesley each see more and more instances of pomade acne , or breakouts on the forehead and cheeks induced by way of special pore-clogging hair products. "Smoothing serums, warmth styling sprays, and depart-in merchandise contain silicone-derived parts and oils," they write. "You would not moisturize your face together with your hair serum, would you?" Be wary of hair products that incorporate PVP/DMAPA acrylates, cyclopentasiloxane, panthenol, dimethicone, silicone, quaternium-70, oils, and petrolatum, as they conveniently clog pores.

The satisfactory means to do that is get rid of them from your movements absolutely—that is the road I took. Can't live without your favourite anti-frizz product? Are attempting covering your face before you spray, doing all your hair before your make-up (washing your fingers fully in between), and choosing a coiffure that keeps your hair away from your face.

talk to your meals.

Just cut up some succulent strawberries? Love the way in which your turkey burger smells? Supply it a compliment, even though it's in your head. The primary segment of digestion starts once we suppose starvation or smell meals, Dattner explains. "Most religious and spiritual traditions admire this segment with silence or a prayer of thanks earlier than eating, bringing the intellect far from the cares of the day," he says. Being reward along with your meal is most important for calming your parasympathetic apprehensive procedure, which is in charge for efficient digestion.

When you consume even as you're harassed, unfocused, or in a hurry, this system gets overridden when you consider that your physique is in battle-or-flight mode, activating your sympathetic nervous system. Before I a meal, I say my thanks and face a window, considering the fact that i know this may occasionally hold me calm and concerned with every chunk.

Moisturize.

Moisturize.

I used to be skeptical at first. Why put an oil-headquartered product on my already oily skin ? Esthetician and holistic dead - care specialist Brooke Leidner explains, "if you are missing oil or overproducing oil, applying jojoba oil can aid normalize the skin due to the fact that it can be the closest factor to your ordinary sebum." acne products have the tendency to dry my dead with acids and harsh chemicals, but I also located my dead getting more and more oily once I used them.

"regardless of feeling oily, it's fundamental to preserve the dead hydrated to steadiness the dead 's sebum creation," Leidner says. Are attempting utilising jojoba oil by myself or in an natural and organic moisturizer (my favorite is PurO3, which is made from natural and organic jojoba and pure oxygen). "Jojoba can also be antifungal and antibacterial with the aid of nature," says Leidner. "Of path, every case of pimples is exact."

prime 10 home remedies for pimples that you could try today

Our skin is a mirrored image of our interior wellness. Glowing, beautiful dead shows appropriate care, hydration and a healthy acne diet. Skin ridden with whiteheads, blackheads and different acne suggests oxidative damage, negative diet and hormonal imbalances.

Occasional breakouts and persistent acne plagues tens of thousands of american citizens of all a long time each yr. From moderate to severe, circumstances of acne rationale painful and unpleasant outbreaks on the face, back, chest and even palms. Left untreated, acne can result in diminished self-esteem and scarring.

Alas, many folks choose possibly dangerous prescription medications and topical medicinal drugs over normal home cures for acne. But getting rid of pimples naturally is viable, as is minimizing acne scars.

Moreover to most important oils, appropriate smooth cleansing and appropriate diet, we'll examine the exceptional dwelling cures for acne , together with how you can get rid of unsightly acne and scars.

top 10 home remedies for acne to check out today

every person's dead is exclusive, so preserve in intellect that with no trouble treating pimples breakouts at house requires a multi-disciplinary approach to care and a healthful weight loss program. The house treatments for pimples beneath can be used in combination, nevertheless it's essential to avert the most important mistakes in treating acne :

1. Settling on blemishes

2. Over cleansing with harsh chemicals

three. Believing handiest topical care of the skin is fundamental to battle pimples

four. No longer giving dead the chance to adapt to new care

5. Failing to remain safely hydrated

6. Failing to treating pimples from the within, out

when you to find the right mixture of residence treatments for pimples, continue along with your personal application for the first-rate results.

1. Gentle cleansing

getting rid of stubborn acne , blackheads and whiteheads starts with thorough however tender cleaning. Try my recipe for selfmade Honey Face Wash. Dampen dead with heat water, and massage into face and neck. Rinse well and pat dry. Do that every morning and evening and, if needed, after workouts. Refrain from cleansing more on the whole, as this may irritate the dead   and rationale an overproduction of oil.

It facets apple cider vinegar, honey, coconut oil, probiotics and principal oils (like tea tree oil). The honey soothes the skin , the coconut oil helps to combat micro organism and fungus, and the tea tree oil helps to invigorate the dead .

2. Firming

toning is an major step in correct dead   care. It helps to dispose of any residue after cleansing and helps to revive the skin's natural pH phases.

Use pure apple cider vinegar (with the mum tradition) as your evening and morning toner. With a cotton ball, tender over skin paying distinct concentration to lively breakouts and acne   prone areas.

Apple cider vinegar is packed with potassium, magnesium, acetic acid and various enzymes that kill micro organism on the skin . Persistent acne will also be the influence of bacteria and fungi that continue to spread and grow on the surface of the skin .

Three. Therapy Masks

To hydrate and heal the skin , masks should be utilized a couple of occasions per week. Yogurt, honey, cinnamon, foremost oils and other ingredients support to hydrate dead   and fight common explanations of acne .

Yogurt and Honey masks: mix one tablespoon of uncooked honey with one tablespoon of yogurt. Apply to face, paying specific concentration to hairline, jawline and different acne   inclined areas. Loosen up for 10 minutes and gently wipe off with a humid cloth.

Cinnamon and Honey masks: combine two tablespoons of uncooked honey, one teaspoon of coconut oil and half teaspoon of cinnamon. Delicate over face. Preserve faraway from eyes, as the cinnamon may also be an irritant. Chill out for five–10 minutes and gently cast off with damp cloth. Honey and cinnamon used collectively helps to combat acne because of its anti-inflammatory, antioxidant and antibacterial residences.

Add a couple of drops of tea tree oil to both of the masks above for the duration of an energetic acne   breakout. Tea tree oil is viewed one of the most nice dwelling cures for acne.

4. Exfoliate most often (however Gently)

Clogged pores and dead skin make contributions to pimples. (three) It's principal to exfoliate accurately to get rid of the buildup. Commercially on hand scrubs are ridden with chemicals that may additional irritate skin .

DIY scrubs to battle pimples and preserve dead   recent are easy to make and economical. First, you want something that is gritty. Sea salt, brown sugar and floor oatmeal are just right selections. Moreover, you want a base. Coconut oil, kefir and honey are all just right selections.

These bases support to fight micro organism, fungi and Candida overgrowth on the dead   at the same time the textured ingredients aid to unplug pores and remove useless skin .

Mix two tablespoons of the dry ingredient of option with 1–2 tablespoons of the bottom of choice. Rub into skin in a circular motion. Begin on the brow and work your manner down, paying unique concentration to difficulty areas. Dispose of with a humid cloth, and rinse well.

5. Spot deal with

pimples responds well to melalecua, extra traditionally referred to as tea tree oil. It's used across the world as an antiseptic and to treat wounds. Like coconut oil, honey and cultured milk merchandise, it fights bacteria and fungi.

Consistent with scientific study, tea tree oil gels containing 5 percentage tea tree oil could also be as robust as medications containing 5 percent benzoyl peroxide. (4) Researchers do indicate that tea tree oil may fit extra slowly for some participants.

This house relief for pimples asks for you to mix four–eight drops of tea tree oil and one teaspoon of coconut oil or jojoba oil. Dap lightly onto trouble areas. Mild tingling is average. Perpetually use a provider oil, as tea tree oil will also be too harsh when applied directly to skin .

6. Battle micro organism

Holy basil and sweet basil most important oils have been observed to fight pimples prompted via micro organism, in line with a record published in the international Journal of cosmetic Sciences. (5)

on this study, sweet basil oil somewhat outperformed holy basil oil in topical purposes. Holy basil oil tea, or Tulsi tea, supports healthy blood sugar and hormone phases. As these two conditions are linked with acne, ingesting herbal tea everyday will stability hormones naturally, combating pimples from the within out, making this some of the satisfactory move-over residence cures for acne .

Moreover, the tea can be utilized topically as a toner to acne - susceptible or trouble areas. Either sweet basil or holy groundwork most important oils can also be introduced to the masks, cleaner or exfoliating recipes acknowledged above.

7. Moisturize

opposite to widespread notion, acne -susceptible skin nonetheless desires to be moisturized. Using topicals that target drying out the skin tips the dead into producing more oil, thereby growing the acne .

Even as it may be too heavy for some dead , coconut oil is an best moisturizer. A be taught published in Biomaterials found that the lauric acid determined in coconut oil demonstrates the strongest bacterial exercise against acne prompted by way of bacteria. (6)

Coconut oil is without doubt one of the most versatile and healthy oils on this planet. There may be an growing demand for coconut oil beauty merchandise seeing that the lauric acid, antioxidants and medium-chain fatty acids hydrate and restore skin and hair.

As a every day moisturizer, warm ¼ teaspoon of coconut oil in the hands of your hands. Smooth over face and neck. Allow to soak into the skin for five minutes. Gently wipe off extra oil with a dry fabric. The quantity that has been absorbed is your whole skin desires. Any extra may just reason a breakout.

For pimples-susceptible skin and throughout breakouts, it's principal to guard against sun publicity. Ultraviolet rays stimulate pigment producing cells, growing the threat of acne scarring. (7)

industrial sunscreens are full of harmful chemicals that may irritate sensitive skin and acne -susceptible skin . Study shows that coconut oil has an SPF price of 8, as does olive oil. (8) to make use of as sun defense, follow a average quantity to uncovered skin every couple of hours.

Eight. Take a Probiotic complement

bear in mind, combating acne requires each outside cure and an internal healing. Reside probiotics support healthy digestion and immune method functioning, plus improves skin wellness by fighting acne.

Consistent with a contemporary gain knowledge of published in Dermatology on-line Journal, researchers point out that probiotic meals supplements are a promising and trustworthy acne treatment. (9) The be trained suggests that better trials are needed, but the indicators are promising.

9. Take Guggul

For contributors affected by the cystic form of acne, a managed clinical trial has discovered that Guggul dietary supplements (sometimes called guggulsterone) outperformed 500 milligrams of tetracycline via a small margin. (10)

in the gain knowledge of, 25 milligrams of guggulsterone taken twice day-to-day for three months resulted in the reduction of acne , but more importantly, 50 percentage fewer participants had pimples relapses. Researchers noted that sufferers with oily dead replied remarkably better to guggul than others within the study.

10. Devour healthy

As a part of the protocol to treat acne   from the within out, it's fundamental eat meals that don't intent blood sugar spikes that lead to the production of insulin. Focus on leafy inexperienced veggies, berries and clean protein.

Develop consumption of wild fish, grass-fed meat and cage-free chickens. Healthy fats are primary to good dead   wellbeing and treating pimples breakouts at dwelling, so include meals wealthy in omega-3s like wild-caught salmon.

Add zinc-wealthy foods akin to kefir, yogurt, lamb, pumpkin seeds and hen. In line with a latest gain knowledge of released in

BioMed study global, there is a correlation between low zinc levels and the severity of acne.

This learn excited by youngsters and younger adults with acne vulgaris, the variety of acne that is induced by way of infection and clogged pores.

Meals to preclude for acne -free skin comprise hydrogenated oils, gluten, wheat, sugar and traditional dairy. If you need to have your dairy milk, consume uncooked milk, as researchers have located that conventional milk products can make a contribution to acne .

furthermore to conventional dairy, it's principal to exclude known allergens or meals you might have a sensitivity to — fashioned food allergens include gluten, tree nuts, soy, peanuts and shellfish.

dwelling cures for acne   Scars

The enormous majority of participants that get acne will expertise some measure of scarring. During a breakout, on no account decide upon or pop pimples, whiteheads or blackheads.

For 6 –365 days after an acne breakout, keep out of the solar as a lot as viable. If you find yourself within the solar, use an all-ordinary sunscreen to aid decrease the possibilities of acne scarring. Treating pimples scars takes persistence and perseverance.

The sooner you treating a scar, the simpler viable outcome. If scars do strengthen, dot a drop of rosehip seed oil or carrot seed oil on the scars twice per day unless you realize a change in the scar. Coconut oil, lavender main oil, honey and tender exfoliation may also help, relying on skin tone and texture.

ultimate hints for acne

upon getting gotten rid of acne, it's main to stick with a healthy eating regimen, drink plenty of water, hold up with your new skin care routine and change your pillowcase per week.

If you in finding that pimples appears around your hairline, business hair merchandise may be responsible. Shampoo, conditioner, hair spray, gels and mousses contain pimples-inflicting elements, including petroleum, parabens, silicone, sulfates, panthenol and different chemicals.

Are trying my homemade Honey Citrus Shampoo that's void of damaging chemicals and leaves hair gentle and manageable. Follow with a contact of coconut oil or my selfmade Conditioner made from apple cider vinegar and main oils.

Like hair products, make-up and dead care products incorporate constituents that may rationale acne . Fashioned offenders comprise lanolin, mineral oil, aluminum, retinyl acetate, alcohol, oxybenzone, triclosan, parabens, polyethylene, BHA and BHT, and formaldehyde-established preservatives.

Whilst the majority of dialogue above focuses on the face, all of these home remedies for pimples can be used on other parts of the body where acne happens. The first-class residence relief for pimples and getting rid of pimples shouldn't be universal. Fighting pimples naturally requires proper skin care and a healthy food regimen … endurance is required. Persist with the healthful events and results will follow.

Normal acne remedies That Work

Some persons select not to use or take man-made merchandise, even relating to pimples remedies. If so for you, common acne cures could also be attractive.

If your acne is severe, or in case you are developing scars or are susceptible to scarring, it's most important to look your dermatologist. He will produce other remedy advice for you, although you come to a decision not to use conventional pimples treatments.

One thing to hold in intellect is that you just don't ought to shun mainstream remedy in prefer of substitute acne therapies all together.

Many persons use ordinary pimples cures at the side of average treatment. Just let your health care provider know that you're doing so.

Usual acne treatments aren't as good-studied as the extra typical pimples remedies, and there is not any consensus on whether they work good or now not. But there are some normal pimples remedies that maintain some promise.

Exchange Your weight-reduction plan

targeted meals don't reason pimples. So, that you may consume pizza and chocolate without guilt (at least, with out guilt of worsening breakouts.)

but some medical professionals are rethinking the way diet influences our skin . There were a number of reports that appear to exhibit a correlation between eating a excessive-carb weight loss plan and pimples severity.

You can also wish to reduce your intake of high

glycemic index foods (like white bread, white sugars, and many others.) and change these foods with entire grain possible choices, fruits and veggies. It's a healthy diet although it doesn't help your skin to clear, and it may be effortlessly and safely used together with different acne medicinal drugs.

Some researchers additionally suppose consuming various dairy merchandise, like milk, cheese and butter, can make pimples breakouts worse. You might are attempting reducing your intake, notably if you happen to consume plenty of dairy, and see if it has a constructive effect in your skin .

These acne cures may be valued at a try, especially if they simply inspire you to eat a more healthy eating regimen.

Detoxing

Detoxing has come to be very standard. There are numerous special "detox plans" from supplements and teas, to fasting, consuming lemon water or consuming handiest raw foods.

Detox proponents say poisonous buildup inside the body can motive a bunch of specific well being issues, including pimples. The idea in the back of detoxing is to aid the physique rid itself of toxins which have gathered from processed foods, caffeine, and so forth. Believers say the skin will clear as the physique is brought into a healthier state.

There are plenty of medical professionals who believe detoxing is pure hogwash. And at the same time it's actual that the skin is an organ of removing, there isn't but proof that any type of detox eating regimen, tea or supplement can support the look of your skin .

Detoxing does have its believers, although. In case you'd like to give detoxing a are attempting, you should seek advice your foremost care healthcare professional first.

Inexperienced Tea

green tea is a healthy drink loaded with antioxidants. But might green tea keep the important thing to clearing acne?

Although it's too soon to understand for targeted, a number of (albeit small) reviews which have shown topical application of a green tea lotion to be an amazing treatment for moderate to average pimples.

Inexperienced tea has been used in chinese medication for centuries as a alleviation for a lot of illnesses, including acne. Typically in the tradition, a few cups of green tea had been under the influence of alcohol per day. At present, some herbalists go one step extra and recommend making a toner from strong-brewed green tea. There isn't proof past anecdotal evidence that this is necessary for acne, though.

Inexperienced tea extract is a usual ingredient in many skin care merchandise, but many don't contain enough to rather benefit your skin. Learn the constituents and shop around.

• Hidden health benefits of green Tea

Tea Tree Oil

right here's one substitute acne remedy that has some science in the back of it. Tea tree oil is by and large essentially the most good-studied of all typical acne cures.

Some reports have proven it to be as potent as benzoyl peroxide, even though it does take longer to see outcome. Tea tree is a powerful antiseptic and is believed to kill P. Acnes, the bacterium responsible for acne breakouts.

Tea tree oil will also be observed at most average food shops or wellbeing food shops. It is also incorporated into cleansers, soaps, toners, and lotions.

Zinc

ensuring that you are getting ample of the vital nutrition and minerals is important to your well being. In case you have acne, it usually is doubly main to get enough zinc.

Used both orally and topically, zinc may aid slash inflammatory acne. Some topical pimples medicines, like Theramycin Z, include zinc.

You can also get zinc tablets over-the-counter. Zinc can purpose upset stomach and curb the effectiveness of antibiotics. Don't take tremendous-doses of this mineral, seeing that it can reason different wellbeing problems.

That you could get zinc out of your food plan, too. Excellent sources of zinc include hen, beef, pork, peanuts and legumes.

Does Rubbing Alcohol Clear acne?

Rubbing alcohol, that ubiquitous clear liquid at each drug retailer that may be purchased for just a buck or two, has lengthy been a staple in every first aid package. It smells antiseptic and medicinal.

So, it will appear that rubbing alcohol (also known as isopropyl alcohol) would get the skin rather clean. In spite of everything, it is used to clean wounds and sanitize the skin before injections.

Some persons even use rubbing alcohol as a facial toner, hoping it is going to deep clean and resolve acne .

However is that healthful for your skin?

Now not via a long shot.

Rubbing Alcohol Does no longer Clear acne

First, rubbing alcohol isn't an acne treatment. It's not going to solve pimples.

Yes, rubbing alcohol can kill micro organism. But acne isn't induced with the aid of micro organism by myself.

Correctly, there are a lot of reasons that have got to be present for acne to boost. Good acne treatments target all these reasons; rubbing alcohol doesn't.

(And in case you're looking for a approach to heal a popped a pimple rapid, put down that bottle of alcohol! There are higher ways to deal with those buggers: find out how to Heal a Popped Pimple.)

Rubbing Alcohol does not Cleanse or Tone the dead

Wiping your face down with rubbing alcohol could think super cool and fresh, so it's going to appear like you are getting your skin fairly easy. But rubbing alcohol doesn't cleanse or tone the dead , it strips it.

You're much at an advantage utilising a facial wash or cleaning bar to wash the skin , and an astringent for firming.

These products are designed particularly for the skin . They'll do a significantly better job, and in a technique that's gentler and more healthy in your skin.

Rubbing Alcohol Breaks Down the dead 's average Barrier

according to middle for disorder manage, repeated exposure isopropyl alcohol "defats the dead ." because of this, in simple terms, it eliminates the skin 's sebum (or oil).

I do know you're thinking satisfactory! Since you'd like your skin to be much less greasy.

However your skin needs sebum to be healthy. Sebum acts as a common barrier for the skin, and keeps the skin moisturized. Strip it all away and you're skin is left in an unbalanced, unhealthy state.

Rubbing Alcohol will Over-Dry Your skin

Alcohol is majorly drying. Habitually rubbing your face down with it could leave your skin tight, flaky, and aggravated.

And if you're making use of acne drugs, be careful! Adding rubbing alcohol to your skin care pursuits will dry your skin out even rapid.

That is one time you most likely don't wish to "think the burn." if your skin is burning or stinging, it's already feeling the harm from rubbing alcohol.

To fight Oiliness, do this alternatively

There are gentler ways to fight oily skin besides giving your face an alcohol bathtub. In case your skin is still feeling too oily for your liking, you should utilize an astringent to aid decrease excess oil in a soft approach.

For an ideal inexpensive alternative, are attempting witch hazel instead.

Witch hazel is an astringent, cleansing to the dead , and expenses a couple of buck a bottle. You can find it at any drug store subsequent to, sarcastically, the rubbing alcohol.

However recall that with ease taking away excess oil is not sufficient to solve acne . To do that, you'll be able to want an acne remedy product.

Does Turmeric Clear acne and pimples Scars?

Turmeric, that distinct spice that gives taste to curry is a hot new health meals. But can it fairly clear acne and treat acne scars?

Let's take a look at what the science says.

What's Turmeric?

Curcurma longa, as turmeric is botanically identified, is a plant that's native to Asia. It is a relative of ginger, and it has a exclusive spicy smoky flavor.

The basis is dried and powdered to provide us the brilliant golden yellow to orange spice.

It can be generally used in Indian delicacies, and you will see it in the spice aisle of your local grocery store.

Turmeric has been used for centuries in each Ayurvedic and chinese treatment to treat a tremendous array of wellness problems. Traditionally, it is used for some thing from indigestion to arthritis. It is usually been used in folk medicine as a remedy for skin issues like diaper rash, psoriasis, and pimples.

With extra people fitting taken with traditional cures as a whole, it can be not shocking that turmeric is getting a 2d look.

Turmeric Vs. Curcumin

When speakme about turmeric, you'll additionally hear lots about curcumin. Curcumin is a component determined in turmeric.

Despite the fact that there are greater than 300 components in turmeric that have been recognized, curcumin is probably the most commonly studied. The phrases curcurmin and turmeric are probably used interchangeably when speakme about the wellness advantages of the spice.

Turmeric Has a number of wellness advantages

as far as natural cures go turmeric, and exceptionally curcumin, has been studied more than most.

The list of health benefits given to turmeric is lengthy and different.

Turmeric is credited as being an anti-ager and a strong antioxidant. It is indicates promise as a viable treatment for arthritis, diabetes, and Alzheimer's disease. Researchers are additionally learning turmeric for anti-cancer homes.

Both topical and oral turmeric has been studied.

And, even though turmeric is one of the most widely researched herbal relief, we nonetheless have very constrained info as of yet.

Early proof indicates some promise, however far more study wishes to be completed to look precisely what turmeric can do, and how it does it.

Curcurmin Kills acne -inflicting bacteria, In Vitro at the least

as far as acne is worried, turmeric does have some features that makes it valued at a more in-depth seem as a feasible pimples remedy.

Inflammatory acne is, partly, brought on with the aid of bacteria known as Propionibacteria acnes (P. Acnes). This bacterium is a normal resident of the skin ; it doesn't mean you are unclean or unhygienic whatsoever.

This bacterium is fitting more immune to antibiotics which have been used to deal with pimples for many years. So, there may be been curiosity find other antimicrobial dealers to step up and take this position.

Reviews have shown that curcumin, that primary factor in turmeric, kills P. Acnes and does so even better than the acne drug azelaic acid.

This was carried out in vitro, because of this in a scan tube in a lab, and likewise demonstrated on pig's skin .

It wasn't performed on human dead . And easily in view that it really works in a lab does not imply it is going to work the identical on human skin .

More research needs to be achieved on this discipline, but it's a just right start.

Turmeric Has Anti-Inflammatory houses

usually probably the most well-known and well-studied advantage of turmeric is its anti-inflammatory first-rate. There is some indication that turmeric may support reduce the irritation of acne, both when taken orally or used topically.

But there haven't been any colossal scientific trials done, so we relatively do not know for definite what (if any) outcomes turmeric has on acne.

Turmeric Has not Been demonstrated to treat pimples or acne Scars

although turmeric and its constituent curcumin has proven some promise, it has now not been confirmed to aid remedy acne. As of yet, it hasn't been validated to have any influence on any dermatological limitation.

As for acne scarring, some a couple of sources claim turmeric helps fade hyperpigmentation, so it is going to help topically to fade dark pimples marks. There is nothing to recommend that turmeric has any influence on pitted or depressed acne scars.

Still, there's sufficient to maintain researchers watching into this natural remedy.

Topically, Turmeric may just motive skin infection

this is a element about turmeric that we're designated about: it could possibly reason contact dermatitis.

Some humans enhance redness, itching, and blisters after making use of turmeric instantly to the dead . That's obviously not something you need to discover after making use of turmeric in every single place your face!

Recall, simply because turmeric is a traditional substance would not guarantee it can be strong, or even safe, for your skin .

Take Care—Turmeric Can Stain Your skin (and everything Else)

a further quandary to turmeric is its potential to impart its colour on the whole lot it touches. It is used as a dye in many cultures as a result of this very fact.

So before you go and whip up a turmeric masks, understand that the intense yellow spice can stain your skin , your counter tops, washcloths, towels, and some thing else it is available in contact with.

Methods to add Turmeric to Your pimples dead   Care hobbies

After weighing the pros and cons, you can also come to a decision so as to add turmeric to your acne treatment pursuits. Typically, turmeric is an extraordinarily reliable natural alleviation.

Cook With It

The simplest, and honestly probably the most scrumptious, strategy to get your dose of turmeric is so as to add it to your food regimen. Add it to curries, soups and stews, rice, or steamed greens.

It can be a versatile spice that you can do rather a lot with.

Drink Turmeric Tea

a different technique to up your turmeric intake is to drink it in tea. There are a lot of prepackaged teas that contain turmeric, or that you would be able to effortlessly make your possess with the dried root or powder.

Take Turmeric or Curcumin dietary supplements

Curcumin or turmeric dietary supplements are one other option. Be certain to follow the recommendations on the package. Despite the fact that they're in most cases well-known as riskless, colossal doses of turmeric/curcumin can cause upset belly.

Additionally, you'll want to talk together with your health care provider first before starting on supplements to make sure it is riskless for you to take action. Curcumin can have interaction with exact drugs. Those with gallbladder ailment also shouldn't use these supplements.

Use a Turmeric masks or cleaning soap

rather get your turmeric topically? There are some over-the-counter skin care products that incorporate turmeric (how so much of the spice they without a doubt include although is debatable).

In the event you make a decision to make use of a DIY turmeric mask, test to be certain you won't have a response to the spice before you use it on our face. You can do a patch test by making use of a bit of your DIY concoction to the criminal of your elbow for your inside arm. Let it set there for a few minutes, then rinse off.

Monitor your skin for redness, inflammation or rash for the subsequent 24 hours. Not having a reaction to your arm does not assurance you is not going to have a reaction on your face; but if your arm does emerge as annoyed you will understand unequivocally to now not apply it to your face.

The patch experiment may also show you precisely how much staining you can get from that specified recipe. You can be ready to observe your stain removing method if the turmeric does flip your skin orange.

Understand which you could increase a sensitivity to turmeric over time. So it is possible to have a response despite the fact that you've used the spice for your skin earlier than with out a situation.

Turmeric can also be drying to the skin , so take care in case your skin is already feeling dry. And, of course, ask your dermatologist earlier than trying any turmeric products, whether pre-made or handmade.

You'll be able to Get the satisfactory acne-Clearing outcome from validated acne medicines

whether or not you decide to make use of turmeric or now not, your satisfactory choice for clear dead is to make use of a confirmed acne remedy. You can get better and extra constant results with these cures alternatively than an herbal relief.

If you want support with therapy, make an appointment with a dermatologist. There are many pimples therapy options to be had with the intention to give you the results you want.

Does Olive Oil Heal acne Scars?

Acne can be so tremendously frustrating -- not simplest the breakouts however what it does to your skin afterwards. Lots of persons feel just like the darkish spots, uneven skin tone, and scarring is even worse than the acne themselves.

So, it's best normal to want to eliminate those, and quick. However, as exotic as olive oil could also be in other applications, it's not a just right cure for pimples scars. It's now not a therapy for scars at all, relatively.

Olive Oil, historically and in these days, Is Used as a skin therapy

Olive oil has a protracted, wealthy historical past. It's no longer only used as a food. Humans have additionally utilized it to their hair and skin for hundreds of years.

As a folk remedy, olive oil is used as a skin moisturizer and hair oil. It's a normal ingredient artisan soaps, lip balms, sugar scrubs, and bath oils. It acts as a lubricant, giving the products satisfactory "slip" and a gentle think.

Olive Oil is not going to Heal pimples Scars, although

however as lovely as that sounds, we ought to be sensible about what olive oil can relatively do. Making use of olive oil to the dead won't heal acne scars.

Those dark spots left over as a pimple fades are called post-inflammatory hyperpigmentation. It's the dead 's natural, albeit stressful, response to a wound (in this case, an infected pimple). The discoloration can't be light with no trouble by using moisturizing with olive oil.

The same goes for depressed or pitted scars.

Olive oil cannot transform the skin and intent it to rebuild itself.

Olive Oil Can Clog Your Pores

there's another motive you will not wish to rub olive oil onto your face: it can clog your pores. Most sources list olive oil as slight to reasonably comedogenic. Whilst you're using it in the hopes of improving acne scars, which you can clearly be making your acne much worse.

In my opinion, i love ordinary cures. However simply considering the fact that something is traditional does not make it a greater alternative to your skin . In this case, olive oil isn't a good pimples scar remedy. You can get much better outcome, and be so much happier, with a established scar healing.

For darkish pimples Spots, do this

There are treatments you can use to aid fade post-inflammatory hyperpigmentation. Over-the-counter merchandise that contain glycolic acid or niacinamide can be worthwhile, specifically for minor discoloration. For deeper discoloration, prescription treatments like topical retinoids and azelaic acid are a greater wager.

For Pitted Scars, do that

Depressed or pitted scars (typically known as pockmarks) are, lamentably, more difficult to get rid of than put up-inflammatory hyperpigmentation. Olive oil won't do something for pitted scars. You won't in finding any OTC lotions or lotions which can be potent for them both, regardless of claims through all those "scar treatment" creams.

As an alternative, you'll wish to talk to your dermatologist about what can also be completed about your scarring.

There are legit tactics that may delicate the dead and scale down scars. Laser remedies are most commonly used to treat acne scars. Your dermatologist would also advocate dermal fillers to "plump up" the depressed field leaving the skin , albeit temporarily, extra delicate and even.

These are simply among the scar remedy options, however there are various more to be had (this article provides you with a rundown of probably the most most customary: Your Scar medication choices.) talk together with your dermatologist to get the news on which cures could be the fine fit for you.

Will Coconut Oil Clear pimples or acne Marks?

Coconut oil is having its heyday. And why now not? No longer most effective does it make a first-class cooking or baking oil (you have got Got to check out it in pineapple upside-down cake), coconut oil has found it is manner into our beauty routines as good.

You should utilize it as a body balm, moisturizing hair treatment, cheap eye makeup remover.

However many sources declare coconut oil can deal with pimples and erase acne marks. Is it relatively that powerful?

Coconut oil will have antimicrobial houses.

Coconut oil is lovely effective, simply. Coconut oil is excessive in many free fatty acids, certainly lauric acid.

Lauric acid has traditional antimicrobial houses. Reviews have proven that lauric acid can kill propionibacteria acnes, the foremost bacteria dependable for inflicting acne.

Some research has been completed on whether or not lauric acid perhaps used as an pimples treatment. Even though initial outcome look promising, it's still a way off.

Coconut oil itself is not an acne healing, although.

Just due to the fact that coconut oil is excessive in antimicrobial fatty acids, does not make treating acne as handy as rubbing a dab to your face.

To work, the lauric acid has to get into the pore the place it is going to do the job. With a view to do that, the lauric acid need to be put in a car (some thing to give the fatty acid) to the place it needs to be.

This is where sources claiming coconut oil can kill acne -inflicting bacteria are lacking the mark. Even though coconut oil does have fatty acids with antimicrobial homes, the oil itself is not amazing adequate to influence pimples.

Pimples isn't completely brought on by p.Acnes bacteria anyway. You additionally need a healing that will preserve pores from fitting clogged within the first position.

Coconut oil won't do that, in view that...

Coconut oil can clog your pores.

Although many traditional skin care authorities and web pages state coconut oil won't clog your pores, all sources I've observed label coconut oil as medium to high on the comedogenic scale.

In easy terms: coconut oil can clog your pores. If you're susceptible to acne breakouts, commonly applying this oil to your face (or at any place else you get acne) may be doing more harm than just right.

Coconut oil and marks or scars.

Coconut oil can aid moisturize the skin , and make it feel silky smooth. But it surely is not going to repair the skin . Lamentably, it cannot do some thing to fade acne marks or heal scars.

These dark marks left after acne heal are known as post-inflammatory hyperpigmentation. Post-inflammatory hyperpigmentation almost always fades, all by itself, over time.

So, if you happen to've been religiously rubbing coconut oil onto these marks, it may appear just like the coconut oil is fading them. In all certainty, the marks would have faded all on their possess. (those marks no longer fading? There are approaches to treat them!)

Pitted or raised acne   scars will not change a lick with coconut oil. These forms of scars want pro therapies to particularly improve .

As an alternative of coconut oil, do this.

You don't have got to toss your coconut oil. It's a enjoyable, normal addition to your magnificence hobbies (remember, not to your acne -prone areas although). Simply don't pin your hopes on it as an acne   medication.

Alternatively, you can need to take a look at over-the-counter pimples remedies first. Probably the most potent OTC products include benzoyl peroxide.

If OTC products don't give you the outcome you are watching for after eight to 12 weeks, a prescription medication is the next satisfactory step. Your dermatologist or loved ones general practitioner can aid you make an strong acne -busting plan.

Does Aloe Vera Clear acne and Scars?

Aloe vera is a trendy plant remedy for a lot of skin problems. However what about for acne?

Does aloe vera clear acne or get rid of acne scars?

What's Aloe Vera?

Aloe vera is a succulent plant native to Africa. Inside its plump leaves is a pulpy center full of copious quantities of mucilaginous gel.

Aloe vera has been used mostly on all manner of skin irritations. The contemporary leaves can also be damaged off of the plant, the gel squeezed out and applied instantly to the skin .

It can be a wellknown houseplant and can be observed at any neighborhood nursery. But you could have a lot of different options should you'd rather now not grow your own aloe plant.

The plant's gel is used as a base for the over-the-counter aloe gels that you would be able to buy at the store. Aloe vera is used in a plethora of dead care preparations, from cleansers to moisturizers, masks, and more.

Aloe Vera Is an Anti-Inflammatory

there's a excellent intent that aloe vera is used for therefore many skin issues—it has anti-inflammatory houses. That implies that aloe vera can help minimize swelling.

Placing aloe vera on a crimson, swollen pimple can aid scale down tenderness and soreness. Aloe also has wound cure effects, so it may aid heal open pimples blemishes.

Aloe Vera Can Soothe the skin

At some point, you've gotten in most cases aloe gel on a sunburn. Just as aloe soothes the sting of sunburn, it might probably additionally soothe a number of other dead   irritations together with acne.

If pimples treatments are leaving your skin   dry and annoyed aloe vera gel, or a moisturizer containing aloe, will also be specifically important.

Your skin will be more secure, so you can be much less more likely to ditch your pimples medicines.

Aloe Vera may just improve Effectiveness of acne medication medicinal drugs

the benefits of aloe vera may go past just soothing aggravated dead . Some research has shown that aloe vera may boost the effectiveness of acne   medicines.

One study, released within the April 2014 dilemma of the Journal of Dermatological treatment, when put next two groups: one utilizing topical tretinoin and aloe vera gel, the other utilizing tretinoin and a placebo.

The team handled with tretinoin and aloe vera had much less redness, and no more pimples, than those treated with tretinoin alone.

Aloe vera additionally has antibacterial houses. Given that acne is, in part, prompted via micro organism known as propionibacteria acnes, it's speculated that aloe may play an element in reducing these micro organism. This has now not been proven, though. It's viable aloe has no outcome on propioni acnes.

Acne will not solve With Aloe Vera by myself

even though there may be some wonderful preliminary research, we're still some distance from saying that aloe vera is an robust pimples therapy. The study, as of but, may be very confined.

So far, it would not seem aloe does way more than lessen redness and irritation. This, undoubtedly, may also be helpful in soothing inflammatory pimples.

However pimples isn't brought about by irritation alone.

Additionally it is triggered by means of a buildup of lifeless dead cells, over-lively oil glands, hormones, and even genetics. Aloe vera will not do anything for these reasons.

What's more, each pimple begins off as a blocked pore. Aloe vera does not hinder pores from becoming blocked, so in the end it is not going to discontinue acne from developing.

Aloe Vera can't Erase pimples Scars but could help With Hyperpigmentation

Aloe vera cannot repair depressed or pitted pimples scars. These are brought on by a lack of skin tissue. Truly the only solution to improve the looks of those varieties of scars is with dermal fillers. That you would be able to ask your dermatologist for help in treating pitted acne scars.

However aloe vera could support fade submit-inflammatory hyperpigmentation, those darkish acne marks left after acne have healed. That is due to a constituent in aloe vera referred to as aloin.

Aloin is a compound that's naturally observed in aloe vera gel. It's a depigmentation agent, so it helps to lighten darkish areas on the skin.

And, on the grounds that aloe vera reduces inflammation, it should maintain publish-inflammatory hyperpigmentation from constructing within the first position.

Should You Add Aloe Vera to Your remedy movements?

Aloe vera isn't a indispensable addition to your pimples treatment program. But, when you have infected acne, or your skin is aggravated and dried out from pimples medictions, aloe vera merchandise could also be worthy.

One factor to do not forget is every aloe gel is one of a kind, so learn the ingredient listings. You may be amazed to search out that the "aloe" gel you may have bought comprises little or no aloe vera.

Just don't count on aloe vera to be a miracle remedy—it's no longer. You'll nonetheless have to use a traditional acne therapy remedy, like topical retinoids or benzoyl peroxide, to fairly see development of your skin.

Most significantly: If you're utilising any prescription acne medications, ask your dermatologist before including aloe vera gel to your acne healing hobbies.

Will a Cinnamon masks Clear your pimples or pimples Scars?

Natural remedies had been making a colossal comeback over the last several years. There is some thing very pleasing about growing something from ordinary elements, along with your own two hands, and using that remedy to repair a obstacle.

The trick is understanding which cures are dependable and strong, which are not, and if the main issue you're trying to repair must be treated via a health care professional instead.

In the case of acne treatments, the cinnamon mask makes me uncomfortable on a quantity of stages.

I do not care if herbal-alleviation-lovers blast me for this, but a cinnamon mask is not an powerful acne remedy. And i do not think it can be all that excellent to your skin, both.

Cinnamon masks can irritate your skin .

First, let's simply look on the security issues. Rubbing cinnamon onto your face could irritate touchy skin facial dead and cause a foul rash called contact dermatitis.

Are there persons who use cinnamon masks with none issues whatsoever? Yes, sure. However there are a lot of people who tried them and had been rewarded with a red, aggravated face. You quite cannot be definite how your skin will react, so you have got to ask your self if it is rather worth the hazard.

Doesn't cinnamon kill micro organism?

Even if you should utilize cinnamon on your skin, with none in poor health-results, the next query is will it solve your acne?

There don't seem to be many excellent, stable reports on the results that cinnamon has on bacteria and even much less on the outcomes it will have (or won't have) on acne .

Some sources say cinnamon has antibacterial traits, there's no evidence in any respect that cinnamon kills the acne-inflicting micro organism propioni acnes.

Besides, acne isn't completely triggered by way of micro organism. Just knocking it out isn't enough to maintain breakouts from forming.

So the science really isn't at the back of this one.

Using a cinnamon mask isn't going to resolve an lively case of pimples, unluckily.

Alternatively of cinnamon, try this.

Even though cinnamon is not that acne treatment silver bullet you're watching for, it can be no longer all bad information. There are other choices available in the market as a way to be just right for you.

Looking for a therapy for infrequent pimples?

In case you best get the occasional blemish, you don't need a every day pimples treatment per se. Do not rely on cinnamon or that other oft-recommended (however pretty horrible) spot remedy, toothpaste. As a substitute try some of these verified treatments to banish that zit: Breakout 911: Heal That Pimple quick

needing an potent healing to get pimples beneath manage?

Despite the fact that I are not able to propose any effective kitchen therapies for acne , i will do the subsequent nice factor for you --

present up some cure choices that relatively do work. Yes, some of them require a shuttle to the dermatologist, however on the end of the day if your skin is obvious, won't it be worth it? Robust acne   healing options

Honey has been used as a food and in normal remedy given that ancient instances. It has been credited with healing, antioxidant, and moisturizing homes, and even today is utilized in skin care and beauty preparations.

Now not simplest is that this sticky stuff scrumptious, honey is an awfully elaborate substance containing proteins, amino acids, vitamins, enzymes, and minerals.

However it's the antimicrobial motion of this sweet treat that have individuals speculating that honey is also the excellent medication for pimples.

It's cheap, all-typical, and also you normally have it to your pantry correct now.

Honey may just scale down bacteria.

As far as dwelling therapies go, honey is in most cases one of the crucial great-studied. And it does have some optimistic outcome.

Honey from in every single place the arena has been shown to have antiseptic, antimicrobial, and anti-inflammatory properties. Some reviews have proven designated types of honey may battle nasty bugs like pseudomonas and staph, including MRSA.

In some circumstances, honey is getting used as a wound and burn dressing, with good results. It's additionally being verified as a medication for other skin issues like dandruff, psoriasis, ringworm and athlete's foot, and contaminated wounds.

Store-purchased honey isn't the identical.

There are numerous types of honey. Clover honey is distinct from acacia honey. And uncooked honey is different than purified, pasteurized honey. Any antimicrobial recreation (or lack thereof) is going to be affected by the form of honey used.

Studies have proven is there is a large range of honey's effectiveness, depending on the type. Essentially the most largely studied, and the one shown to have the absolute best antimicrobial satisfactory, is Manuka honey.

The stuff you purchase on the grocery retailer in the bear-formed bottle? It commonly doesn't measure as much as its medicinal cousin.

Honey is a typical product, so it's ever-altering. The medicinal fine of the honey goes to be affected by many extraordinary factors – the forms of vegetation the bees had access to, where on the planet the hive was located, the time of year it was once made.

There are so many variables you can't just make a blanket assertion that all honey is good for pimples (or something else for that matter).

Micro organism isn't the one acne -causing element.

Even though honey have been to wipe out acne -causing micro organism, it still wouldn't leave your skin breakout-free. Bacteria is only one piece of the acne puzzle.

Pimples can be prompted with the aid of over-active sebaceous glands, and skin cells that can't shed competently. These create blocked pores, making a pleasant dwelling for propioni bacteria to flourish. Even though you deal with the micro organism, these other causes are nonetheless there.

So, as fantastic as it might be, honey by myself gained't solve a case of acne.

As a substitute of honey, do this.

Honey continues to be an effective ingredient. It's a enjoyable addition to your DIY skin care.

Go ahead and take a look at a honey masks – it'll leave your skin feeling smooth, smooth, and refreshed. (however actually I wouldn't try these strategies to sleep in it, unless you wish to have a enormous ol' mess for your pillow, sheets, to not mention your hair.)

As for treating pimples, you have plenty of options. Start off with over-the-counter pimples cures. Give it a few weeks to work.

If these simply aren't reducing it, you've Got a lot of prescription choices as well. So, put in a call to a dermatologist.

Then all you need to do is relax and patiently wait until your acne medicines start to work. Would I endorse a first-rate cup of tea with a big spoonful of honey?

Can an egg masks particularly clear acne ?. Picture: Riou / Getty snap shots

by way of Angela Palmer - Reviewed with the aid of a board-licensed medical professional.

here's a recipe that's been around for a while: the egg mask.

There are a few unique recommendations for this replacement pimples alleviation. Some say use the egg white most effective; different say use simply the yolk. Nonetheless others recommend beating the whole egg together, both white and yolk.

The inspiration is all of the identical, though: observe the uncooked egg to your skin, let set unless absolutely dry, and rinse thoroughly.

Proponents say it will possibly lessen gigantic pores and clear acne.

What does the science say?

An egg mask is not going to solve a case of acne.

Utilising uncooked egg, whites or yolk, as a masks won't make acne go away. Even though the skin may think softer, or even cleaner, after you employ this masks, long run it's not going to resolve breakouts.

There are as a rule a couple of factors why humans feel egg has acne-clearing advantage. First, as it dries it tightens on the face (it will get fairly, quite tight) a lot within the same way a clay facial mask would.

It could appear like because it tightens it's drawing impurities and gunk from the pores. In all actuality, raw egg is not cleaning out the pores. Certainly your skin quite often feels cleaner. Egg isn't "cleansing" all those tiny microcomedones from the skin. And it's these micro-breakouts that finally grow up to be be breakouts.

Eggs yolks do incorporate diet A, but no longer in a technique so one can discontinue breakouts.

One other rationale eggs are most likely idea to have acne - clearing talents is seeing that they are high in vitamin A.

Many of our most powerful acne remedy medications are derived from nutrition A. This involves topical retinoid drugs, like Retin-A

And Retin-A Micro (tretinoin), Differin (adapalene), and Tazorac (tazarotene), and the oral medicine isotretinoin.

So, it does appear like you'll be ready to skip the center man, so that you could converse, and put a food high in nutrition A directly in your skin alternatively and get the equal outcome.

Here's the change, although: while these drugs are derived from diet A, they aren't the same vitamin A you in finding in foods like eggs. They have got been created in a lab to have a distinctive outcome on the dead , specifically a keratolytic effect (which means it makes your skin peel).

Eggs, certainly, wouldn't have the identical effect in your skin .

Eggs may at some point play a position in the best way we treat pimples.

Apparently, some studies were executed on eggs and ways they is also capable to support treat pimples. These aren't your average eggs you opt for up at the grocery store, though.

Researchers have immunized laying hens with Propionibacteria acnes, the bacteria largely liable for inflamed acne breakouts. Antibodies were accrued from the yolks of eggs, laid by means of the aforementioned immunized hens, which had anti-acne properties.

Despite the fact that this was all performed in a lab, now not on human skin , the thought is might be sooner or later these anti-acne antibodies can be utilized to deal with acne.

Instead of an egg mask, do that.

There's no harm in utilizing an egg masks for a fun DIY facial.

  Simply would not have excessive hopes that it is going to utterly clear your skin .

(there is a small risk of contracting salmonella from raw egg, so do take care not to get it into your mouth. I would recommend pregnant females keep away from this altogether, to be secure.)

If you are quite watching for a excellent treatment to your pimples, you will be higher of making use of a tried-and-actual cure. Here are some choices to get you started.

Should you were to feel everything you learn, a vegetarian or vegan food regimen could be a healthy, average, and sure-fireplace strategy to clear your acne . A vegetarian would not devour any style of meat—no pork, pork, fowl, or seafood. So, can doing that hinder breakouts? Probably. According to a few reviews, pimples may be linked to a high amount of animal protein within the weight loss program.

The link Between Meat and acne

there is a protein-difficult within the human physique referred to as mammalian goal of rapamycin elaborate 1 (mTORC1).

MTORC1 is accountable for healthy cell growth and performance. Which you could say that mTORC1 tells our cells what to do and learn how to do it.

Some researchers suppose that mTORC1 turns on the pathway (or chain response) for the body to create acne breakouts. MTORC1 is activated by vitamins and minerals, principally amino acids like leucine. Meat, like pork and bird, occurs to be naturally high in leucine. But it's now not just meat that contains leucine—unique proteins preferred with vegetarians, like whey, egg, and soy are additionally high in this amino acid.

Here is the place it will get fascinating: mTORC1 can also be "overstimulated" by high amounts of leucine. When the mTORC1 pathway is over-activated, it could possibly impact sebum (or oil) construction, skin phone growth, and irritation. Leucine has an extra trick up its sleeve: It acts as a constructing block for the sebaceous glands to create sebum (or oil). All of those factors are linked to acne development.

The over-activation of mTORC1 may additionally expand androgen hormones. Androgen hormones are recognized to be a big participant in acne progress. Plus, over-activation of this mTORC1 pathway has already been linked to distinct ailments, like form-2 diabetes and cancer.

The mTORC1 pathway is a very elaborate one, although.

So, to thoroughly flesh out the theory that meat consumption actually contributes to acne breakouts, extra study desires to be carried out. Thus far, there is no such thing as a smoking gun. Finally, eating a steak excessive in leucine does not automatically imply you'll get away with acne.

Backside line: the jury is still out on this one. There hasn't been ample study executed on the link between meat and pimples to say conclusively come what may.

Will Going Vegan aid Clear acne?

Like vegetarians, vegans don't devour meat, but vegans also steer clear of any meals that come from an animal—dairy merchandise, eggs, and many times honey.

There is some proof that dairy performs a role in acne development and severity. Dairy products were shown to in all likelihood set off breakouts in sensitive humans. Skim milk and cheese appear the definitely culprits. Identical to with meat, these contain excessive quantities of leucine. Some reports recommend that the hormones in milk might also play a role. Others point to the excessive levels of insulin-like development factor-1 (IGF-1) in milk.

Apparently, IGF-1 additionally stimulates mTORC1.

It is essential to understand that dairy consumption hasn't been proven to rationale acne in people who commonly have clear dead . As a substitute, milk may just cause a worsening of current breakouts for some people.

Other animal-established meals like eggs, lard, and honey have not been proven to have any have an effect on on acne   progress, or they haven't been studied.

Again, a vegan food regimen hasn't been proven to clear acne . Reducing back on dairy products could reinforce breakouts in some circumstances for some humans. But a fully vegan food regimen doesn't appear to be necessary in any case.

I'm Vegetarian or Vegan and nonetheless Have pimples! Why?

Diet may just play a function in acne   development, however it's likely a aiding player as a substitute than the famous person. You can have the healthiest weight loss plan ever, vegetarian, vegan, or or else. That you could eschew sugar, cut out all junk meals, devour handiest natural and organic meals... And nonetheless have pimples. We all know humans who eat meat and dairy merchandise and certainly not get so much as a pimple, and there are dedicated vegans who battle with pimples every day.

How our diets work on the physique and skin may be very complicated and not fully understood. We do recognize there is not a direct one-to-one hyperlink between any sort of food and acne breakouts. So, undoubtedly, it's now not as simple as pronouncing "meat explanations acne ," or "dairy makes you get away." drinking a pitcher of milk doesn't assurance a breakout tomorrow; consuming two slices of William Maxwell Aitken will not reason two acne to show up.

For some individuals, designated meals could have an effect on acne progress and make existing breakouts worse. For others, though, diet would not seem to influence acne somehow.

If fitting, or staying, vegetarian or vegan is principal to you, there is no motive why you should not (as a minimum where acne is worried). There are various one-of-a-kind causes why humans choose a plant-centered eating regimen, be it for well being causes, to shed some pounds, or moral beliefs. But if you are a card-carrying carnivore since a switch to vegetarian fare completely when you consider that you're hoping to clear your skin , you can probably be disappointed. Some individuals could see an growth of their skin, however the risk that with ease altering your eating regimen will make pimples completely disappear is slim.

So, How Do I Get My acne   underneath manage?

Already treating your pimples and looking to provide your remedy slightly enhance? You now recognize that going vegetarian or vegan is not a imperative step to take to clear your skin . Which you could get pimples underneath control without primary dietary changes. Persons accomplish that at all times.

For moderate pimples and blackheads, over-the-counter acne merchandise may be all you want. For the most strong OTC outcome, recollect utilising a product that includes benzoyl peroxide or salicylic acid. Use it for roughly 10 weeks and see when you get the improvement you wish to have.

In case your acne is reasonable to severe, or for those who've tried OTC products for a time with none outcome, skip the over-the-counter merchandise (they are doubtless no longer strong sufficient). As a substitute, make an appointment with a dermatologist. There are plenty of prescription medicines, each topical and oral, that can support clear your skin.

Simply don't forget, dietary changes could aid support your skin in some cases. However the quickest and most effective solution to clear acne   is with a validated acne   treatment.

Celebrities rave about it. Countless Youtube movies extoll its virtues. And a rapid web search pulls up 1000's of pages of understanding announcing it will probably do the whole lot: scale back blood strain, rev up metabolism, soothe heartburn, and banish warts.

What is this amazing product? Apple cider vinegar, or ACV, to these within the comprehend.)

Now, I really love the stuff. It makes a yummy French dressing. And, due to the fact that I consider homemade magnificence merchandise are tremendous enjoyable, I once whipped up an apple cider vinegar hair rinse and an apple cider vinegar toner.

However can apple cider vinegar resolve acne ? No.

In fact, there are numerous causes why you must not use apple cider vinegar for acne . Here are only a few:

it could actually burn your skin .

Many sources claim that on the grounds that apple cider vinegar is usual, it has no part effects. Now not genuine.

Should you put apple cider vinegar for your skin , undiluted, it can reason a nasty burn. Even ACV diluted in water is robust ample to burn skin that's touchy to it.

It's not mighty.

ACV proponents say apple cider vinegar works on acne by means of killing bacteria. Additionally they surmise that, in view that it's acidic, it eliminates dead dead cells and unblocks pores.

The bottom line is there haven't been any excellent experiences executed on the consequences apple cider vinegar can have on acne .

So even as it is going to manipulate micro organism in the lab, it may well have another outcomes on micro organism on the skin.

Extra importantly, apple cider vinegar contains acetic acid, now not the acne -fighting salicylic acid or glycolic acid. It simply is not going to work the equal method.

It stinks.

Apple cider vinegar smells loopy dangerous. Some folks liken the scent to sweaty health club socks.

Keep in mind the apple cider hair rinse and toner I advised you about previous? I used them as soon as and that used to be it. I could not recover from the scent.

Admittedly, this can be a personal factor. But if you're in any respect scent-sensitive, you'll not like the aroma.

Drinking it would not work either.

There were more reports done on the effects of apple cider when taken internally. But again, none exhibit that it has any clearing outcome on pimples.

The About.Com alternative medication expert has a quality article that lists probably the most feasible wellness advantages of apple cider vinegar: Apple Cider Vinegar: What You need to comprehend.

Take into account, although, that taking apple cider vinegar internally can also have facet effects. It can erode the enamel of your enamel, and if taken undiluted in big portions can rationale injury to your esophagus, stomach, and different constituents of your digestive tract.

Rather of utilising ACV for acne, are trying confirmed acne cures alternatively.

If you're studying apple cider vinegar for pimples it is doubtless you have tried other acne cures without outcome and are determined for an answer.

I do know when you consider that i have been the place you're right now. And if I thought ACV was real a miracle medication for acne , believe me, i would be shouting it from the rooftops.

However apple cider vinegar just isn't an pimples medication. Given that i need you to get real growth, i'm suggesting you forgo the ACV.

As a substitute of apple cider vinegar, try this:

• For moderate acne, are trying an over-the-counter cure like benzoyl peroxide.

• For reasonable to extreme acne, you can need a prescription treatment. A dermatologist can support advance a therapy plan with a purpose to give you the results you want.

• If one remedy does not work, don't quit. There are remedy options on the way to give you the results you want.

If you are in any respect serious about aromatherapy, substitute medication, or even naturally-situated skin and hair care merchandise, you're ordinarily acquainted with tea tree oil.

Tea tree oil is obtained from the leaves of the Melaleuca alternifolia plant, a woody shrub that is native to Australia. Traditionally, this oil has been used for dead infections, fungal infections (similar to athlete's foot), ulcerations and different wounds.

Today, it is usually a customary ingredient in soaps, body washes, tub merchandise, and shampoos.

Many supply say it can be an potent acne cure -- however is it fairly?

Tea tree oil does have antimicrobial houses.

Tea tree has been shown to have antimicrobial properties, which is commonly why it's a popular common alleviation for treating acne . It is idea that tea tree helps kill Propioni acnes bacteria, which can be responsible for acne breakouts.

More reviews must be completed on the effects tea tree oil has on pimples.

Unluckily, just a few small reviews have been accomplished, so the genuine outcome tea tree oil has on acne is still uncertain.

One study, evaluating tea tree oil with benzoyl peroxide, determined tea tree extended both infected and non-inflamed acne breakouts. It wasn't fairly as amazing as benzoyl peroxide, and it did take longer to peer growth. However tea tree did not cause dryness, peeling, and flaking because the benzoyl peroxide did.

A extra recent gain knowledge of located 5% tea tree oil generally elevated pimples when compared to a placebo. Despite the fact that the outcome of each reviews look promising, way more research desires to be completed before tea tree oil may also be listed as a verified acne healing.

If you are dedicated to average therapies, tea tree oil is also valuable.

Committed to utilising simplest natural remedies on your skin?

Then tea tree oil is probably your pleasant option for a common, replacement acne cure remedy.

Tea tree important oil may also be purchased at any ordinary meals store, but should be diluted before making use of to the skin. Most aromatherapist suggest diluting tea tree oil in a service like coconut oil or sweet almond oil, however beware! These oils can clog your pores and make acne worse.

You may also decide it's easier to buy a skin care product that includes tea tree oil, as a substitute. In the event you go this activities, learn the ingredient record and prefer person who has tea tree oil because the active ingredient.

Tea tree products are excellent used as spot remedies for the occasional pimple.

Demonstrated acne therapies are still your excellent alternative.

In case you have extra than just the occasional blemish, and your pimples is extra chronic, tea tree oil isn't probably the most amazing option. You'll be able to be better off making use of a tested OTC acne product like benzoyl peroxide, or getting a prescription remedy from your dermatologist. That is above all true for stubborn or extreme acne .

Already utilizing prescription acne cures? Be certain you ask your healthcare professional earlier than you comprise tea tree oil merchandise into your hobbies.

Does making use of Toothpaste to your acne fairly Work?

Toothpaste is most often idea of as an low-priced spot cure for blemishes, however that is one home comfort you don't want to take a look at.

I know some men and women swear toothpaste dries up their acne speedily, in reality most people will to find the toothpaste leaves their skin pink and aggravated. Without doubt not what you need to do on an already crimson, swollen blemish.

Where Did This notion Come From?

The idea to make use of toothpaste as a spot therapy is on the whole considering that many forms of toothpaste incorporate triclosan. Triclosan is an antibacterial ingredient that's delivered to lots of our personal care items like cleaning soap, deodorant, and physique wash.

Triclosan simply kills micro organism. It is truly a original addition to pimples remedy products, despite the fact that as a preservative and no longer an lively ingredient.

Some studies have found that triclosan can kill propionibacteria acnes, the bacteria that causes pimples. However, it needs to be formulated in a distinct manner to try this. Simply striking any random product containing triclosan, toothpaste, for illustration, isn't going to do the trick.

Toothpaste Can Burn or Irritate Your skin

this is the biggest reason to forgo the toothpaste trick - besides being not going to really work, toothpaste will most often irritate your skin.

Don't forget that seventy five percentage of my pupils that tried the toothpaste on their pimples? More than half of them stated the toothpaste irritated their dead .

(lots of the others mentioned toothpaste did not do a darn thing for their pimple.)

Toothpaste wasn't supposed to be utilized to the skin, specifically the tender skin on the face. Using toothpaste on an already infected pimple can purpose more redness and infection.

Many unfortunate souls have developed a chemical burn after making use of toothpaste to a zit. Your skin could be feeling sore for days in a while. Backside line: Toothpaste can make your pimple look worse as an alternative of higher.

Alternatively of Toothpaste, try this

If you're looking for a option to make a big blemish heal rapidly, are attempting an pimples spot healing as an alternative. These products incorporate benzoyl peroxide, salicylic acid or sulfur, all of which is able to aid reduce redness and speed healing.

Pimples spot therapy merchandise are milder in your skin than toothpaste ever will probably be, and they're cheap to buy. You'll discover many spot cures at your regional drugstore for not up to

$10. Of direction, if you're already seeing a dermatologist in your pimples, ask him/her earlier than making use of any spot medication.

I normally begin off my skin care courses by means of telling my scholars I want to hear all of their most burning acne cure questions. Inquire from me anything! I tell them. Perpetually, at this point, anybody asks, "Is it actual that urine clears pimples?"

After the requisite display of shock and disgust from the leisure of the class, everyone cheerfully gives their take on how best to apply pee to the face.

Given that, it appears, there are a lot of versions of this hobbies.

Some say you have to take a youngster's urine-soaked diaper and lay it across the acne -prone skin. Others say you should utilize your own urine, however only from the first-morning pee. There may be additionally this debate: dab person acne or go hog wild and observe it to your whole face?

I've not yet met a man or woman who has simply tried it (besides for anonymous posts on the net and third-hand bills about a person's sister's first-rate pal's cousin.)

Can urine clear acne ? No.

Regardless of what many say to the opposite, there's certainly no scientific proof that urine does whatever to treat acne . No formal studies were completed on the outcomes urine has on acne. I would venture to bet that's partly attributed to the truth that now not many persons would volunteer for that one.

So, where did this suggestion come from?

Traditionally, some cultures have used urine to treat more than a few health issues. Even at present, some alternative healers espouse the healing houses of pee and use urine cure as a remedy for a kind of well being issues.

(observe that there is not any proof that urine is an amazing therapy for any wellness obstacle.)

Even the old method of urinating on a jellyfish sting is not medically sound. Our About.Com First help expert says pee does not fairly work for jellyfish stings.

What your pee is made from.

Urine is virtually absolutely, greater than 90%, water.

Water, most likely, doesn't treat pimples.

The following greatest constituent in urine is urea.

Here is where it will get exciting -- urea surely does do some good things for the dead . It is a humectant, this means that it helps preserve dry skin moisturized. It's also an exfoliant and may help hold lifeless cells from collecting on the outside of the skin.

Many dead care merchandise contain urea -- cxamine the labels. Don't worry, the urea used in skin care merchandise is synthetic. There's no urine, human or in any other case, in there.

Perhaps now you are considering which you can make your own urea, without cost!

But to be amazing, you need far more urea than is naturally located in urine. So, an genuine skin care product is still the excellent technique to get it.

As for urine being acidic and drying up acne, that's now not accurate both. If that have been the case, vinegar can be a fab acne medication (it's now not) when you consider that it's rather more acidic than urine. Urine is an extraordinarily vulnerable acid. Nothing about it might dry up a pimple.

Urine is a waste product.

The predominant thing to don't forget, though, is that urine is a bodily waste.

Placing pee on the face is solely plain icky.

Contrary to standard perception, your urine is not sterile. There are low phases of bacteria even in a healthy person's pee.

That does not mean it is toxic, though. I am a mother, as a consequence i've been soaking wet in someone else's pee on a couple of occasions with definitely no ill effects. Heck, there are reports of people who survived practically unsurvivable circumstances by using consuming their own urine. (don't try this, incidentally. Drinking urine is not going to clear pimples both.)

alternatively of urine, do this.

I proudly admit that i'd are trying urine medication if I proposal it would clear my skin. I have been close to desperate enough to do it, too.

But we should thank our fortunate stars there are different pimples cure choices that work, with out the yuck factor. Listed below are some to get you began:

just don't forget to give any medicine a lot of time to work (about 3-four months). And when you've got questions or need help, ask your health practitioner.

Don't seem to be you comfortable you quite don't have got to lodge to placing pee for your face?

Top 4 principal Oils for acne

Tens of millions of american citizens endure from acne . Correctly, an estimated 70 percentage–ninety percent of young adults, each ladies and men, endure from pimples. And latest stories show that the incidence of adult female acne has extended.

Yet so many can't seem to find a remedy that actually works! Most turn to prescription drugs or chemical cures — investing within the modern day "pimples-curing resolution" that has instantly hit the market and can reply all of your prayers.

Actually that these products often incorporate harsh chemical compounds which have aspect effects or just don't work at all. That's why I suggest you seem to traditional, house cures for acne which were used for thousands of years. These cures comprise most important oils that tackle the root of the difficulty and are soft on the skin .

Correctly, one essential study observed that tea tree oil was once practically six occasions more effective than the placebo in treating mild to reasonable pimples! My prime four predominant oils for acne will nourish your skin and combat the reasons of acne naturally, with out adding insult to damage with dead -stressful products.

Why Use foremost Oils for acne?

Persons of all a long time are plagued by occasional breakouts and continual pimples plagues. Acne can intent painful and unsightly breakouts on the face, chest, again and even palms. When it's left untreated, acne can result in diminished self-esteem and scarring.

The fundamental causes of acne incorporate clogged pores, bacteria, extra oil construction and dead skin . Different reasons, such as hormones, weight loss program, stress and exact medicinal drugs, corresponding to corticosteroids, androgens, beginning manipulate tablets and lithium, might also worsen pimples.

Why do so many, teens in particular, endure from acne? Good, it can be as a result of genetics, changing hormones phases, stress or dead -demanding endeavor. For illustration, friction from sporting activities apparatus and backpacks can irritate the skin and cause pimples breakouts on the chin, brow, jawline, neck, chest and again.

Nevertheless it's most important to understand that harsh chemicals and over-the-counter or prescription drugs can intent additional inflammation — exacerbating the obstacle. Most important oils have the power to kill micro organism on the skin naturally. Some main oils for acne, corresponding to lavender oil, soothe and safeguard the skin from irritation and stress.

But acne isn't simply affecting teenagers; contemporary experiences exhibit that the incidence of adult female acne has multiplied. This can be due to stress, hormonal imbalances and sleep deprivation, in line with a 2014 be trained carried out in Brazil.

predominant oils for acne , akin to lavender and clary sage, have the ability to alleviate feelings of stress and anxiety, battle insomnia and sleep deprivation, and balance hormone stages. They're also tender on the skin and have a quantity of advantages that go past combating acne and promoting skin wellness.

top four main Oils for acne

1. Tea Tree

Some tea tree oil advantages incorporate its antimicrobial and antifungal residences. Over-the-counter acne therapies containing tea tree oil at the moment are greatly on hand, and evidence indicates that they are a usual option among men and women who self-treat their acne .

A scientific evaluate of the efficacy, tolerability and talents modes of motion in regard to the remedy of pimples with tea tree oil states that tea tree merchandise lessen lesion numbers in sufferers with pimples, have tolerability phases which can be just like different topical cures, and have antimicrobial and anti-inflammatory movements which might be associated with the healing of acne. (2)

A 2007 be taught means that tea tree oil is an strong medication for mild to reasonable pimples vulgaris. Sixty sufferers had been divided into two companies — one staff used to be handled with tea tree oil and one was the placebo. The participants had been followed every 15 days for a interval of forty five days. The response to therapy was once evaluated by using the total pimples lesions counting and acne severity index.

The results of the learn showed a gigantic difference between tea tree oil gel and placebo within the growth of the whole acne lesions depend, as tea tree oil was 3.6 occasions more robust than the placebo. In regard to total pimples severity, tea tree oil used to be 5.8 occasions extra potent, proving that tea tree oil serves as an powerful and ordinary medication for slight to average acne . (three)

to make use of tea tree as an main oil for acne , add 2–three drops to a smooth cotton ball and observe topically to the field of trouble. Tea tree can be added to your everyday face or body wash — corresponding to my Face Wash for clean skin — or it may be brought to a sprig bottle full of water and spritzed on the face or body.

2. Lavender

Lavender oil has profound advantages in your skin on the grounds that of its antimicrobial and antioxidant traits. It soothes and nourishes the skin — treating acne, treatment dry dead , and decreasing the looks of dark spots and scars triggered by means of acne . Different lavender oil advantages include its capability to shrink stress and anxiousness which can be associated with acne breakouts in adults and its therapeutic homes that toughen your quality of sleep, thereby promoting healthful and radiant skin .

A be taught released in the Journal of the scientific organization of Thailand found that lavender oil presents a relaxing effect when inhaled. Twenty volunteers participated in a learn that investigated the effects of lavender oil on the primary apprehensive system, autonomic nervous process and mood responses. The outcome published that lavender oil induced significant decreases of blood stress, coronary heart rate and skin temperature. The contributors characterised themselves as extra secure and refreshed after lavender oil inhalation.

stories advocate that stress and acne are linked, explaining why men and women on the whole expertise pimples flare-united states of americain instances of expanded stress and anxiety. This can be considering that cells that produce sebum (the oily substance that mixes with useless skin cells and bacteria to clog hair follicles) have receptors for stress hormones.

Researchers suppose that an develop in pimples may be due to larger stages of sebum that are produced in occasions of stress; therefore, lavender important oil serves as a strong tool since of its stress-lowering capabilities.

to use lavender oil to alleviate emotions of stress that may set off the creation of sebum, diffuse 5 drops of oil at residence or apply topically to the wrists, back of neck or temples. Lavender most important oil also has antibacterial properties and can be used straight on the skin to battle acne.

Three. Clary Sage

An most important ester reward in clary sage, called linalyl acetate, reduces skin irritation and works as a ordinary relief for acne and skin irritations. It additionally regulates the production of oil on the skin , a aspect that is generally related to breakouts. Clary sage additionally curbs the development and unfold of bacteria, alleviates feelings of stress and anxiety, and helps hormonal balance.

Stress is a fundamental reason of acne in grownup ladies due to the fact that it's related to an increase in the phases of the stress hormone cortisol. A 2014 be taught published within the Journal of Phytotherapy study determined that the inhalation of clary riskless oil has the potential to slash these cortisol phases through 36 percentage. Researchers concluded that clary sage has a statistically colossal outcome on reducing cortisol stages, and it has an antidepressant effect, bettering mood and combating anxiety.

A up to date be taught published in Advances in Dermatology and Allergology determined that clary sage principal oil is an energetic traditional antimicrobial agent. After checking out the efficacy of clary sage on more than one drug-resistant bacterial stains, clary sage oil used to be active in opposition to bacteria that leads to dead   infections that can result in acne breakouts or skin irritation.

To increase typical treatments for anxiety and stress, diffuse 5 drops of clary sage oil at dwelling. This additionally helps with restlessness and insomnia — two conditions related to acne breakouts. To kill micro organism that is clogging your pores and causing acne , follow 1–3 drops of clary sage oil to the field of predicament. It may be applied with a clean cotton ball or via diluting it with jojoba or coconut oil after which massaging the combination into the skin .

Four. Juniper Berry

Juniper berry fundamental oil has typical antibacterial and antimicrobial advantage, making it one of the vital trendy normal remedies for combating dead   irritations and infections. It serves as a house comfort for acne and helps gorgeous skin. It also has detoxifying and stress-reducing homes that guard the body against toxins that lead to pimples.

A 2005 learn released in Pharmaceutical progress and technological know-how states that juniper berry oil has antibacterial activity that serves as an anti-acne topical solution. The antimicrobial recreation of juniper berry oil was once studied as it made contact with acne vulgare. When used with neat software or after dilution with service oils, juniper berry primary oil confirmed promising anti-acne recreation; the changes didn't cut back the antibacterial endeavor of the oil.

a number of reports point out that juniper berry main oil is a strong antibacterial agent that fights pimples when used topically. This is due to distinctive compounds, together with alpha-pinene, p-cymene and beta-pinene.

Use juniper berry as an ESSENCIAL oil for acne by using applying 2–three drops topically to the field of main issue. For touchy dead , dilute juniper berry with coconut or jojoba oil earlier than topical application.

how to Use ESSENCIAL Oils for acne

Topical Use — The first-rate means to use ESSENCIAL oils for acne is to use 2–three drops topically to the field of drawback. These oils are dependable for neat or direct application, but they may be able to even be mixed with a carrier oil equivalent to jojoba or coconut oil.

Actually, when utilising coconut oil for skin wellness, you'll notice surprising advantages. Coconut oil hydrates the dead   and is able to penetrate your skin   on a deeper degree than your normal product for the reason that of its low molecular weight and the way in which it bonds with proteins.

Jojoba oil is also a priceless provider oil that enhances skin wellbeing by way of working as a protectant and cleaner. It's wealthy in iodine and fights damaging micro organism development that leads to breakouts. It may well pace up the remedy approach and minimize skin lesions, too.

Face Wash for Clear skin — This face wash is full of probiotics to invigorate the skin and kill acne-inflicting bacteria. Combine the following ingredients:

• 1 tablespoon coconut oil

• three tablespoons honey

• 1 tablespoon apple cider vinegar

• 20 drops tea tree oil

• 2 capsules of are living probiotics

combine the parts collectively and blend with a hand blender. Then pour the blend right into a convenient bottle and store it in a groovy location.

Another strong face wash recipe is my easy home made Face Wash that leaves the dead refreshed, hydrated and clean. The major oils and coconut oil work collectively to kill micro organism at the same time providing vitamins and minerals and hydration to your skin .

Ordinary acne Scar medication — For a common pimples healing for scars, make a paste by way of mixing the next elements:

• 2 teaspoons uncooked honey

• three drops lavender oil

• three drops tea tree oil

• 3 drops frankincense oil

Wash and dry your face, then apply the paste and let it take a seat for an hour earlier than rinsing off.

Soap Bar for skin Hydration — To hydrate and soothe your skin , try my do-it-yourself Lavender soap bar. Now not most effective does it kill micro organism on the skin that rationale acne, but it eases your mind and brings on emotions of peace and contentment.

viable aspect results

These 4 ESSENCIAL oils for acne are safe and amazing. Take into account that a bit of goes some distance, so making use of 2–three drops on the dead   must do the trick.

When you have touchy dead , dilute the ESSENCIAL oils with a service oil before applying topically. Additionally, avoid exposure to direct sunlight when treating acne with principal oils. The UV rays could make your skin   more sensitive and could result in skin irritations or redness. If making use of any of these main oils causes skin infection, do not use that oil; try a gentler oil like lavender as a substitute.

The Worst acne   home therapies you didn't know

looks like every body has a few acne   home cures that have been passed down from family participants or examine on a internet site someplace. Amazing or no longer, acne house therapies stay standard.

Honestly, when you have more than simply an occasional pimple, most acne   dwelling remedies aren't going to have an considerable outcomes for your skin . You'll keep your self various disappointment, frustration, and (in some cases) cash, via seeing a medical professional about your acne first.

That said, many folks like making use of acne   dwelling treatments. Are any acne   home therapies truely useful? Listed here are the satisfactory (and worst) pimples dwelling cures.

Replacement cures

If the traditional route is where you're coming from while you believe acne   dwelling cures, you're ordinarily interested by substitute cures.

For those who come to a decision to head this route, take some time to educate your self. Most substitute remedies have now not been commonly studied.

Also, be wary of any manufacturer looking to promote their "miracle" acne healing.

That mentioned, some alternative cures (like tea tree foremost oil, zinc, and inexperienced tea extract) have proven promise as acne dwelling cures.

"Kitchen" treatments

Many people love mixing up their own handmade masks. It's a fun pastime. A lot of books and internet pages have recipes for handmade pimples "treatments."

could the key to clear skin rather be proper in your own kitchen? Ordinarily not. If simple kitchen materials worked well, the acne medicinal drugs of in these days would in no way have been developed.

That's to not say there are no benefits to these handmade dead care preparations. They can make your skin feel softer, and are an inexpensive but decadent option to pamper your self.

Simply use common sense when making kitchen facial masks. Many general acne house cures call for lemon, garlic, cinnamon or cloves. When applied to the skin , these can result in contact dermatitis.

OTC treatments

Over-the-counter remedies aren't most often what come to mind when humans consider pimples house cures, however they're without doubt essentially the most potent. Observed at drug outlets, dead   spas, and a few department stores, OTC therapies are easy to search out and most commonly inexpensive.

If you like the notion of excessive-tech acne home therapies, you could want to take a look at the Zeno pimples Clearing gadget. At the same time it's no longer low priced, many people find it works well to curb infected pimples. Zeno pimples Clearing gadget works by using heating the skin , killing the micro organism that factors inflamed blemishes.

So far as pimples dwelling cures go, OTC therapies will provide you with the most bang for your buck.

• compare prices for Zeno

Toothpaste

even as some individuals swear it works for person acne, toothpaste is not going to clear a case of acne .

Many toothpastes incorporate triclosan, which is supposed to kill dangerous breath germs. Triclosan is also an ingredient in some acne   therapy products.

But toothpaste additionally comprises other ingredients that may irritate the skin when left on for long periods of time. Who wishes to annoy an already inflamed zit?

Skip the toothpaste and usc an acne spot therapy alternatively.

Urine

This has to be the most fascinating, if not somewhat demanding, of all acne home remedies. Each person has heard some variation of it: Take a baby's moist diaper and practice it to the face, or use your own urine first thing within the morning.

Folks swear this works. But have you ever ever talked to anyone who truely tried it? Didn't believe so.

There is not any evidence that urine of any type clears pimples, so there is not any need for you to check out this alleviation for yourself (thank goodness).

Is it ok to wear make-up with pimples? 6 matters you can do to restrict Your make-up from inflicting acne

Most teen girls and grownup women who endure from acne enhance a form of affection-hate relationship with their make-up. You depend on it to aid duvet up acne acne that make you believe self-mindful.

However, if you're no longer careful make-up can without a doubt create extra of the very blemishes you are attempting to conceal.

How can you make certain your make-up isn't sabotaging your efforts to clear your skin ? These six tips will support avoid makeup from breaking you out.

1. Not ever sleep to your make-up.

Each night time before mattress, make it a factor to absolutely but gently get rid of all traces of make-up out of your face and neck. This minimizes the chance that the make-up will clog the pores, and in addition eliminates filth and excess oil that built up for your skin in the course of the day.

No need to scrub on the dead . All you rather want is a smooth cleanser and your fingers or a tender washcloth.

After cleansing, consider to apply those acne remedy medications in case you have them.

2. Pick makeup labeled noncomedogenic.

Noncomedogenic makeup does now not contain materials identified to clog the pores. And decreasing the amount of pore blockages is a good place to begin when treating acne .

If you have very slight comedonal pimples, commonly your breakouts will support just by way of changing to noncomedogenic makeup.

3. Easy your applicators frequently.

Half of the fight in opposition to blemishes is lowering the amount of acne-causing bacteria for your skin -- and make-up brushes and applicators are bacteria magnets.

Wash all makeup brushes with antimicrobial soap at least once every week. For a quick, mid-week sanitization, completely spray your brushes with with isopropyl (rubbing) alcohol and wipe extra alcohol and makeup off with a clean paper towel.

Disposable make-up applicators are a excellent substitute, principally if you're tremendous busy and in finding it rough to seek out time to wash your brushes.

4. Select powder-centered makeup rather of liquids.

Despite the fact that liquid make-up offers higher insurance policy, many have an oil base. Without doubt no longer anything you wish to have to position for your acne inclined dead .

Alternatively, bear in mind a powder-situated make-up. They think lighter on the skin, and they have the introduced benefit of serving to to soak up extra oil.

Should you rather love liquid make-up, that's good enough. Simply be certain it can be a just right match for blemish-inclined skin. It should be oil-free and noncomedogenic.

5. Are trying switching brands.

In case your pimples appears to aggravate after wearing makeup for a number of days in a row, you might have considered trying to take a look at another manufacturer. Exact makeup formulations, even those labeled noncomedogenic, can purpose breakouts in sensitive individuals.

If this appears to be the case for you, are trying one other company. Your skin would tolerate one higher than one other.

6. Go bare each time feasible.

Leave your face make-up-less at the least a few times per week. Permit your skin time to breathe and heal.

If you happen to do not feel secure going make-up-free all day, cleanse your face as quickly as you get residence.

This will provide your skin a couple of hours each night to go naked.

Make-up on my own mainly doesn't intent a full-blown case of inflammatory acne, so just keeping your skin naked isn't going to be ample to clear up your skin . The hints above are a excellent foundation for the pimples therapy plan on the way to create real improvement for your skin .

If you are now not already using an pimples healing medicine, whether OTC or prescription, it is time to . These will aid you get blemishes underneath manage, and most you should use alongside together with your make-up.

Chiefly, are attempting to not get discouraged. Discovering what works in your skin is traditionally a topic of trial and error. But with patience and time, your skin can heal. And you could suppose confident with or with out your make-up.

5 pimples therapy Myths Debunked

there are numerous acne cure myths in the market, setting apart reality from from fiction can be hard. Is your favourite pimples treatment tip grounded simply?

Delusion: You must Vigorously Scrub Your skin every day

reality: individuals with acne generally tend to fairly scrub their face, trying to deeply cleanse the skin and get that "squeaky-clean" feeling.

Washcloths, cleansers with abrasive constituents, and coarse scrubs aren't always the nice selections for skin with acne . As an alternative than aid, they can rationale infection that exacerbates infection and worsens breakouts.

Your skin wishes to be dealt with gently to curb friction and irritation. Do not excessively rub or scrub your skin . This is specifically genuine if in case you have inflamed breakouts.

Fable: Sweating Will Cleanse Out Your Pores

reality: despite the fact that it scems like sweating cleans your pores, it quite does nothing to clear pimples. And, for those who aren't cautious about showering immediately after getting sweaty, it will probably in reality lead to an increase in breakouts.

See, your skin has two extraordinary forms of pores: your sweat pore (referred to as the sudoriferous pore) and your oil pore (or sebaceous pore).

Blackheads and acne develop in the oil pore. Sweat, nonetheless, comes from a fully distinct pore. So, sweating will not push blackheads and blemishes from the dead .

The great solution to get rid of these pore-clogging plugs of oil and particles is to have them extracted by a skin care reputable. Preserve them from coming back by way of making use of an acne treatment mediation every day.

Recreation is nice for your physique, but it surely's no longer quite going outcomes your skin .

Fable: Use super Drying dead Care products to Banish Oil

fact: Oily skin generally is a bother, but utilising ultra-drying skin care merchandise isn't the high-quality approach to go.

Your skin wishes some oil to be healthful. Over-drying your skin will lead to issues of its own, like uncomfortable tightness and cracking. To not point out that peeling, flaking skin would not appear all that great both.

The trick is to dispose of extra oil with out stripping your skin of every viable drop. The excellent way to take action is use a foaming cleanser that leaves your skin feeling smooth, but not excessively tight and dry.

If your skin nonetheless feels too greasy for your liking, an astringent can aid dispose of additional oil. But have an understanding of that simply putting off extra oil out of your skin is not going to clear acne.

Acne isn't completely caused with the aid of excess oil. Different explanations are at play here, like hormones, distinctive pimples-causing bacteria, even your genes. Simply drying out your skin with products isn't going to alter these other explanations.

Fable: To Clear acne quick, Use a variety of Topical remedy and Use It most of the time

fact: it can be tempting to slather on pimples medicinal drugs at each possibility, but doing so is not going to heal acne any rapid.

Correctly, using too many acne medications, utilising them too ordinarily, or making use of an excessive amount of at one time can truly harm your skin. Rather of getting the clear skin you had been hoping for, you'll be able to be growing immoderate dryness, peeling, redness, and inflammation.

Constantly comply with usage instructions on all pimples medicines cautiously. Don't forget, it'll take time to look results, so you need to be sufferer. If after using over-the-counter acne treatments for several months there's no noticeable growth of the skin , speak to your health practitioner.

Myth: there is Nothing you can do about acne

reality: today many cure choices are available to strengthen acne. Cures incorporate topical lotions, oral drugs, and more.

Whether or not your acne is mild or extreme, if you're a teen or an adult, there are treatment options available with a purpose to be just right for you. Don't hesitate to name your dermatologist to study what healing choices will probably be most mighty in remedy your skin .

Acne is just not anything you must undergo via. Nearly each case of acne can also be effectually controlled with time, persistence, and persistence.

4 major pimples skin Care Steps

good skin care is a vital part of your pimples therapy movements. With just a few simple skin care "DOs," you'll be well for your technique to healthier dead .

Do take just right care of your skin.

A radical and constant dead care activities is step one in getting your pimples under manipulate. A just right skin care movements will encompass cleansing, exfoliating, frivolously moisturizing, and applying healing merchandise. A good skin care pursuits isn't just for the face; it will help body acne too!

Above all, don't fall into the habit of over-cleansing your skin. Cleaning too most commonly can strip the skin , and will not support pimples to clear any rapid. Twice everyday cleansing, morning and night time, is more than ample to clear your skin of filth, make-up, sweat and extra oil.

• daily dead deal with pimples-prone skin

• Exfoliation cures

• how one can care for physique acne

Do follow cure merchandise over whole affected subject.

Most pimples cures work with the aid of reducing pore blockages and acne -inflicting micro organism. Making use of them all over the face (or different physique areas) that is affected by pimples will support zap acne earlier than they show up, clearing the skin way more quite simply than spot medication only.

• don't simply Spot deal with Your pimples

Do let dead dry wholly after cleansing, earlier than making use of your medications.

Even the tiniest little bit of moisture left on the dead whilst you apply your anti-acne merchandise can set off infection. Ideally, you must wait 20 to 30 minutes after cleansing before applying your topical acne medications.

• Dry skin is an effective thing... In this Case

Do use best noncomedogenic merchandise.

It pays to understand what you are striking in your skin. Some dead and hair care merchandise block pores, developing comedones and contributing to a type of pimples called pimples cosmetica.

Make certain everything you set in your skin, from moisturizers to makeup, is labeled noncomedogenic. Noncomedogenic merchandise don't incorporate pore-clogging ingredients, and are a have to if you're susceptible to breakouts.

What Works, What would not , and how to Use Them to Heal Your acne

we have all had that exceptionally worrying pimple that we wish we could speedily zap away. In a technique, which you could with an pimples spot healing.

What Are acne Spot remedies?

Spot remedies are over-the-counter pimples merchandise that aid to heal these pesky acne. In contrast to different varieties of acne remedies, they're supposed for use handiest on present blemishes.

Some spot treatments are left on overnight; others dry clear so you can put on them out throughout the day.

That you may even to find tinted spot cures that aid camouflage breakouts.

Whichever product you decide upon, make sure to read and comply with the usage guidelines.

Spot therapies Can aid Heal character acne , but will not totally clear up acne

Spot remedies are most important for persons who simplest succumb to the occasional zit right here and there (if that describes you, you're so lucky). For those of us who battle with more accepted breakouts, spot therapies aren't going to be as particularly as helpful.

In view that spot treatments aren't applied over the whole face, they is not going to remedy a case of pimples. For that, you would want one more form of healing.

If your acne is moderate, an over-the-counter pimples product possibly ample. However for extreme pimples, you have to get your self a prescription medicine, both topical or oral. These medications, like BenzaClin, Differin, or isotretinoin aid stop breakouts before they .

That you can nonetheless use spot remedies to help character acne heal more rapidly, even while utilising these acne medicines, provided that your dermatologist offers you the go ahead.

Opt for a Spot remedy Containing robust constituents

there are such a lot of spot cures to be had, from bargain drugstore finds to high priced chic brands.

 It particularly doesn't matter which you decide on, so long as it includes a verified acne -fighting active ingredient.

Essentially the most effective spot treatments will incorporate this kind of:

Benzoyl peroxide

It's the most robust OTC acne medication round. Benzoyl peroxide helps lower irritation and makes the pore an inhospitable location for acne-causing micro organism to cover. It can be drying, although, so best use it a couple of times everyday, max.

Benzoyl peroxide can bleach out fabrics, so take care around your towels, sheets, and clothing.

FYI – do not follow a benzoyl peroxide spot treatment over (or below) Retin-A (tretinoin). Tretinoin breaks down chemically when utilized with benzoyl peroxide, so it will not be as strong.

Salicylic acid

Salicylic acid is a beta hydroxy acid. It helps filter gunk that's trapped within the pores. It might also can dry up pustules (acne with white heads).

Sulfur

Sulfur is an additional ingredient that dries out pimples and helps shrink infection. Like benzoyl peroxide, sulfur can be drying to the dead .

Ice

despite the fact that it can be not a natural spot therapy, it needed to be included on this record. It gained't simply heal blemishes any rapid, however icing down enormous pimples can support ease redness and swelling, and makes them feel less sore.

Ice works pleasant on those monster acne   beneath the skin, known as nodules, rather than pustules. The other spot remedies don't work actual well on nodules anyway.

Pay attention of these Spot cure errors

Spot cures could be a worthy addition to your pimples treatment activities. But you'll be using them incorrectly and now not even realize it.

Utilising them too usually.

Nearly absolutely everyone are responsible of this one. Due to the fact that we want that pimple to depart tremendous speedy, we douse it with spot cure at every possibility.

However using any spot medication product too traditionally (and in the event you're making use of it greater than twice a day, you're using it too normally) will dry out the skin. And the one thing worse than a pimple, is a dry, red, flaking pimple.

Using "spot cures" not intended for the skin .

We've all heard of those oddball pimple remedies – Windex, toothpaste, garlic. If any of those bizarre cures fairly worked all that well, we'd all be utilizing them. Actuality is, these varieties of cures don't work, they usually would particularly irritate your skin

.

Utilizing spot remedies instead than a average acne remedy medicine.

Don't forget, spot cures won't resolve your skin. They simply work on person acne which are already visible.

To get really just right outcome, you have got to discontinue breakouts before they even start. This requires daily use of an acne medication remedy, even on areas which can be clear, to hold them clear.

And if your ordinary acne cures aren't doing enough to preserve you breakout-free, it's time to up the ante. Utilising OTC merchandise? Don't forget a prescription medicine. Already using a prescription medication? Let your dermatologist recognize you're now not blissful with the results. You may must change to a further treatment.

The goal is to get your acne cleared to the factor that you just're no longer having to fear about making use of a spot cure in any respect.

Acne treatment pointers in skin of colour

acne is arguably essentially the most customary skin situation throughout all skin tones. But it might probably reason distinct troubles in dead   of colour -- from dark spots and skin discoloration, to sensitivity to acne remedies.

Treating pimples in dead   of colour requires

here are some acne medication recommendations certainly in your skin form.

Ethnic dead   varies in tone from mild to very deep brown, depending on the quantity of melanin found.

Melanin is the protein pigment dependable for coloring the dead , hair, and eyes. It is usually the pigment that darkens the dead because it tans. Darker skin contains bigger quantities of melanin than lighter skin .

When treating acne in skin of colour, special care ought to be taken. It is ordinarily (wrongly) believed that darker skin is tougher than it's lighter counterparts. Really, brown skin may also be very touchy, and have got to be handled very gently.

Are you sure it's acne ?

Ingrown hairs are particularly normal, above all if your hair grows in curly. Ingrown hairs can look remarkably like acne -- with crimson bumps and whiteheads. The change is these are prompted by means of the hair growing out of the follicle improperly.

Ingrown hairs are treated otherwise too. (not sure if what you've got is ordinary pimples or a case of ingrown hairs? This text will aid you make a decision: Is it acne or Ingrown Hairs?)

Discoloration and scarring is original.

You do not want your pimples treatments to intent the very discoloration you are trying to hinder and do away with.

They may be able to, in the event that they cause your skin to turn out to be irritated.

Your dermatologist will mostly put you on a curb dose of remedy or have you ever use the medicine a few occasions per week instead than day-to-day, mainly in case your skin already tends to be sensitive.

Whilst all dead colors are at chance for constructing discolorations, brown dead is chiefly inclined considering that of the better quantity of melanin found.

Skin of colour is extra prone to dark spots or patches (hyperpigmentation), lack of skin color (hypo-pigmentation), and scarring. Pimples and unique acne remedies can exacerbate discolorations.

It is in particular ESSENCIAL to hinder making a choice on, squeezing, or in any other case irritating pimples blemishes. Doing so can with no trouble scar any skin colour, but in particular ethnic dead . Darkish skin tones are prone to setting up keloid scars. Keloids are massive lots of tissue that boost after a wound heals. Keloid scars grow better than the original wound.

Extra usually, acne causes submit-inflammatory hyperpigmentation. Post-inflammatory hyperpigmentation (PIH) is the natural response of the dead to a wound, corresponding to a reduce, scratch, or acne blemish. After the wound heals, a darkened spot or patch remains. This patch can variety from very mild and faint to very darkish and apparent.

It is fundamental to note that specified acne medication merchandise can purpose dead discolorations in individuals of color. Any product that reasons dryness or inflammation puts the person at risk for hyperpigmentation, or darkening of the skin.

Distinctive care need to be taken when making use of retinoids equivalent to Retin-A or Differen gel, benzoyl peroxide, and other such topical remedies. If excessive dryness, burning, or infection happens, inform your surgeon correct away.

You can deal with discoloration.

Hyperpigmentation is essentially the most common criticism amongst individuals of colour who endure from pimples. The discoloration may also be particularly suggested and fashionable. While most hyperpigmentation will progressively fade over time, it can be severe adequate to purpose embarrassment and have an impact on the self-esteem of sufferers.

There are many over-the-counter and prescription lightening creams on hand to aid fade discolorations more swiftly. Some prescription pimples lotions may also help lighten hyperpigmentation whilst remedy breakouts. You great resolution is to speak to your healthcare professional. He or she will be capable to recommend proper merchandise to make post-inflammatory hyperpigmentation disappear.

Individuals with brown skin often forgo sunscreen; nonetheless, normal sunscreen use may just support darkish spots to fade more quickly. Many dermatologists to find sun exposure increases fading time. If in case you have hyperpigmentation spots, every day application of a noncomedogenic sunscreen with SPF of as a minimum 15 could also be worthy.

Select your hair products carefully.

Surveys have shown just about 1/2 of all acne sufferers with ethnic skin use pomade, or different oils and ointments, for his or her hair. Greater than 70% of those sufferers developed pimples on the forehead. Oil-based hair products can comfortably block pores, developing pimples breakouts. Pomade-caused acne, or acne cosmetica, consists of blackheads, whiteheads, and normal "bumpiness" alongside the brow, temples and hairline.

Once the usage of oil-established hair products is stopped, acne comfortably clears. Nevertheless, many persons find hair pomades are a necessity considering of dry scalp, dry hair, or to support make hair manageable. If that is so, avoid making use of the product where it could possibly are available in contact with the brow or temples. Surgeon Susan Taylor, creator of "acne Vulgaris in people of color," recommends making use of pomade as a minimum one inch behind the hairline, or making use of only to the ends of the hair. Use as little product as possible to get desired influence.

Dry or "ashy" dead is customary amongst darkish dead tones. If you are inclined to acne, opt for your moisturizing products carefully. Exact lotions and lotions, reminiscent of cocoa butter, can clog pores and make acne worse. Consistently opt for gentle, oil-free moisturizers which might be labeled noncomedogenic.

See a medical professional for aid getting your pimples beneath manipulate.

Topical retinoids are a primary line healing. Azelaic acid may be a further remedy alternative

over-the0counter products may fit when you have very moderate breakouts

tips on how to opt for an powerful OTC acne cure Product in your acne

acne is characterized with the aid of the presence of acne , blackheads, and whiteheads on the skin. It customarily impacts the face, neck, chest, again, and/or upper fingers of victims. Acne varies in development from very slight to enormously severe.

Over-the-Counter acne treatments for mild acne

slight acne can also be treated at home with over-the-counter acne remedy products. If possible, it is first-rate to start remedy during this stage.

Moderate pimples approach you'll be able to see blackheads, whiteheads, or milia. You can even have some papules and pustules, however they is not going to be too serious. Slight acne will also be extensively elevated whilst you utilizing the proper OTC remedies. Here are a few options for treating slight acne .

Benzoyl Peroxide

one of the crucial customary acne cures on hand, benzoyl peroxide is discovered in cleansers, lotions, and lotions. It really works through killing Propionibacteria acnes, the bacteria dependable for acne breakouts. Benzoyl peroxide additionally helps unclog pores and reduces irritation of the skin . Benzoyl peroxide is offered over the counter in strengths from 2.5% to 10%.

Some common over-the-counter benzoyl peroxide merchandise comprise: Proactiv, Benzaderm Gel and various regular or store company benzoyl peroxide creams

Sulfur and Resorcinol

Sulfur and resorcinol are as a rule found collectively in acne merchandise. Resorcinol helps hinder comedones by means of putting off buildup of lifeless skin cells.

Sulfur has been used for greater than half of a century to treat pimples, despite the fact that precisely how it works remains to be uncertain. Collectively, these materials also shrink excess oil. Resorcinol and sulfur are on the whole used in strengths of 2% and 5%-8%, respectively.

Some usual acne healing merchandise containing resorcinol and sulfur are Clearasil Medicated Blemish Cream, Clearasil Medicated Blemish Stick, and Rezamid Lotion.

Salicylic Acid

Salicylic acid works by means of correcting the abnormal shedding of dead cells, serving to the dead to shed useless cells extra effortlessly. In this approach, salicylic acid helps slash the number of pore blockages, preventing breakouts. Salicylic acid works notably good for those with blackheads and whiteheads. It's found in over-the-counter cleansers, lotions, and medication pads. The average strength is .5 to 2%.

Merchandise containing salicylic acid comprise Oxy merchandise, Noxzema Anti-acne Gel, Noxzema Anti-acne Pads, Stridex pads, and Dermalogica Medicated Clearing Gel

Alcohol and Acetone

Alcohol and acetone are also utilized in combination in lots of products for greasy skin forms. Alcohol is an antimicrobial and may fit to cut back acne-inflicting micro organism. Acetone gets rid of excess oil from the skin . Collectively they support cleanse excess oil from the dead , reducing the quantity

Of pore blockages. Alcohol and acetone are determined frequently in toners, astringents, and cleansers.

Utilising Your Over-The-Counter remedies

at the same time it can be tempting to treat breakouts with many healing merchandise immediately, doing so would intent inflammation of the skin .

Most acne   treatments dry the skin to a degree, so overuse of these products would motive immoderate dryness, peeling, and redness. You may desire to start with a single acne treatment product, and slowly add extra if wanted. This is above all true if your skin tends to be sensitive or effectively aggravated.

Non-inflamed pimples

To acquire the quality outcome viable, you have to first comprehend your skin. Non-infected acne, which is characterized with the aid of blackheads and milia (whiteheads), typically responds good to salicylic acid merchandise. With a wash or cleaning pad. If after a number of weeks of medication you don't seem to be seeing seen growth you can also add a salicylic acid lotion, provided you aren't experiencing excessive dryness or infection.

Infected acne

for many who are inclined to get infected acne, benzoyl peroxide is an effective therapy to start with. Benzoyl peroxide lotions and lotions will also be discovered at just about every drug retailer. Apply the lotion as directed for a few weeks, after which add a benzoyl peroxide or salicylic acid wash if needed. Once more, extra merchandise must be delivered best if you're now not experiencing excessive dryness or inflammation.

Finding What's right For You

There are additionally complete pimples regimens or "kits" available over-the-counter that contain cleaner, toner and lotion. The merchandise in these kits most of the time incorporate a combo of acne -fighting elements, and might aid take the guesswork out of constructing a everyday dead care movements. These regimen programs do not always work better than products you buy separately, however some humans decide on them when you consider that of their ease of use.

A part of the fight in treating pimples is finding merchandise that work for you. You can also have to test with a number of therapy products before finding person who improves your acne, so try to not get discouraged.

If, after a few weeks of treating your acne with over-the-counter merchandise you don't seem to be seeing growth, do not hesitate to contact your medical professional.

There are more OTC acne treatment products on the market now than every other time in historical past. This is good news you probably have acne , but results in the query: How do you choose one?

It can be typical to think careworn when looking to wade by way of the ever-developing mountain of acne merchandise. However you can learn the right way to narrow your choices and prefer the most strong OTC acne remedy product for you.

Fully grasp Your options

• Cleansers are self-explanatory. However acne-fighting cleansers range from common cleansers in that they include medications that aid stop acne.

• Toners and astringents are in liquid form. They're applied to acne-affected areas with a cotton ball. Pads (Stridex and so forth) are similar, besides the liquid solution is "pre-measured" for you on a pledget.

• Medicated lotions, creams, gels and ointments are depart-on treatments. Due to the fact that they're on the skin for longer periods of time, these varieties of treatments are in most cases most powerful. However they can be extra anxious to the dead as well.

Prefer a kind

The variety of product you want is dependent upon your skin style.

Super-oily skin? Consider astringents, pads, foaming cleansers, gels, and lotions.

In case your skin tends to be common to dry, non-foaming cream cleansers, alcohol-free toners, lotions, lotions, and (in all probability) ointments are good selections.

You do not must stick to just one medication product. Utilizing a couple of merchandise can also be extra amazing (provided your skin can control it, of path).

Create your own three-step cure pursuits a la carte -- pair a medicated cleaner, astringent, and leave-on pimples healing.

Pick products with exclusive energetic elements for even better results (extra on that under.)

check the energetic elements

narrow down your picks by taking a appear on the energetic ingredients. The most mighty OTC acne remedy merchandise will contain benzoyl peroxide or salicylic acid.

• Benzoyl peroxide is the queen bee of OTC acne cures. OTC benzoyl peroxide products can work well for moderate to moderate pimples.

• Salicylic acid is useful for treating very slight breakouts and blackheads. When used together, these ingredients supply an strong "one-two punch".

• different valuable additions to wait for:

- begin reading these ingredient labels!

- sulfur

- resorcinol

- alpha hydroxy acids like glycolic acid

- tea tree oil

decide on a force

To make issues more complicated, the active elements in OTC acne treatments are available in exceptional strengths.

Salicylic acid comes in strengths from zero.5% to 2%. The most potent merchandise will include 2% salicylic acid. Scale back concentrations are good for these whose skin is without problems irritated, however won't be as powerful.

Benzoyl peroxide is available in strengths from 2.5% as much as 10%. Right here better is not constantly better. A 2.5% benzoyl peroxide can also be just as robust as a 10%, however with much less part results.

So, start with a 2.5% first. You might even see just right things happen. If now not, try a relatively more suitable strength and slowly work your approach up, if needed.

Don't worry About rate

Will that super expensive acne treatment product work better than the pharmacy brand?

Now not always.

How strong an acne remedy is has less to do with fee than it does the materials. For those who particularly love the scent and believe of a boutique-y brand acne product, go for it.

But if fee is a main issue, leisure assured you can get good outcome with a customary product from a discount store. Remember, it can be all about the active elements!

Comprehend When it's time to bring within the massive guns

it would be high-quality if every case of acne could be cleared up simply with a drugstore lotion. Unfortunately, that does not constantly happen.

Understand when it is time to quit on the OTC merchandise. When you are not seeing results after three or four months, put in a name to your surgeon.

Pediatricians and family medical professionals most of the time have tons of experience treating pimples and will also be your first stop. They may be able to treat your acne or refer you on to a dermatologist if needed.

Even supposing OTC products don't be just right for you, a prescription treatment may be just what you need to get your skin back on monitor.

Enhance a four step At-dwelling OTC skin Care hobbies That Works for You

some of the most standard over-the-counter acne merchandise are three-step pimples medication kits. These all-inclusive acne regimens incorporate the whole thing you want – a purifier, toner, and cure lotion. Some even include a bonus mask. Proactiv is usually essentially the most well-known (and arguably most extensively used) OTC pimples treatment package, however there are a lot of others on hand as good.

Your 3-Step acne cure with OTC pimples products

however that you would be able to put collectively your possess three-step treatment hobbies, with some thing products you adore. Incorporating a few OTC products together right into a whole cure events gives you better results than utilizing one just product on my own.

Cheap manufacturers can work as good because the more expensive products, so if saving cash is the motivating element, it's totally best to use discount brands. That you may even use probably the most OTC acne merchandise you have already got available.

Take into account, although, OTC acne treatments rather most effective work for mild acne . If you have average acne to extreme acne, or if you happen to've already used OTC remedies and not using a results, you must see a dermatologist rather. On the flip facet, if you're already seeing a dermatologist for your acne , don't add this to your treatment pursuits except you get approval from your surgeon first.

Competent to construct your own customized three-step pimples program? Head to the dead care aisle (or your skin care stash within the rest room cupboard) and seem for these products.

1

with a cleanser

appear for a cleaner that involves the energetic ingredient benzoyl peroxide (seem on the back underneath the ingredient list). Bonus elements if you get person who includes salicylic acid too.

Rather than the lively ingredient, it particularly does not topic what type of cleaner you opt for. If in case you have oily skin, you'll be able to obviously desire a foaming purifier. A non-foaming cleansing lotion shall be a greater option for you in case your skin tends to be on the dry aspect.

What about those cleansers with exfoliating beads? They're nice too, provided that your skin isn't tremendous sensitive and your acne is not too inflamed. If those beads seem to annoy your skin , bypass them and use a cleaner with out alternatively.

Use your cleaner twice every day, morning and night.

2

decide on a Toner

select a toner that contains salicylic acid and/or glycolic acid. These materials aid exfoliate the skin and unclog pores.

Alcohol-free toners are much much less more likely to sting or burn, and they are not as drying both. Dry or touchy skin ? Certainly get an alcohol-free manufacturer.

A further choice -- these healing pads. (feel Stridex, Oxy, etc). They supply blemish-fighting medication as good, and you do not must pre-moisten your cotton ball. Look forward to skin inflammation, although.

Whichever product you decide on, use twice day-to-day after cleansing, morning and night.

Three

finish with a treatment Lotion

That is the spine of your OTC healing regimen. Pimples cure lotions give you the most bang in your buck.

Seem for a benzoyl peroxide lotion or cream. One of the vital most fashioned brands are Clearasil, Oxy, AcneFree, and so forth. You'll on the whole wish to begin with a 2.5 to 5 percentage force. You could transfer as much as a ten percent strength later, if needed.

Pimples cure lotions don't seem to be moisturizers, and they definitely can dry your skin . If you would like, you need to use an oil-free moisturizer underneath your cure lotion. Observe it first, let it take in fully, after which put your benzoyl peroxide lotion over it.

You are going to use your treatment lotion a few times day-to-day, after cleaning and firming. Don't wash the treatment lotion off.

4

Bonus: Add a mask (not obligatory, but a high-quality suggestion)

A bonus therapy, and one that may aid velocity matters along, is a medicated masks. One of the crucial most necessary: glycolic acid, sulfur, salicylic acid, and benzoyl peroxide.

Masks can support exfoliate (a necessity for maintaining pores from fitting clogged), decrease oiliness, deep cleanse, and make the skin consider softer and smoother. Think of it as intensive treatment on your skin .

Don't go overboard with facial masks and scrubs though, or you could make things worse by way of annoying your skin. A few times a week is just right; everyday is regularly overkill.

Use your masks one to three times per week, in line with the recommendations in your product.

Your At-residence pimples routine

that is all there may be to it! Don't forget, do not fear about the company title; focus on the energetic materials. You need to use anything brand you adore, and you could even mix-and-healthy products from one of a kind manufacturers to create your possess personal acne skin care line. The primary factor is to use your OTC healing hobbies always. Do see a dermatologist if your remedy isn't working after three-4 months, but with success your OTC acne medication pursuits will likely be simply what your skin wanted.

5 Steps to aid You Get the ideal purifier on your acne-inclined skin

Been to the skin care aisle as of late looking for an acne cleaner? Then you have visible the overwhelming alternatives. But don't fear. With a bit of information, that you may opt for the correct acne cleanser for you.

1. Decide on a type of cleanser you adore first-class.

Foaming or non-foaming? Bar or liquid? This rather comes all the way down to individual alternative. All forms of cleansers work equally good, so opt for the one you're most at ease with.

As a basic rule, non-foaming cleansers or cleaning lotions are typically much less drying than foaming cleansers. These are a excellent option if your skin is of course on the dry side, or if it can be drying out because of your acne treatments.

Many persons swear you must never use bar cleansers on the face, but it's fairly ok when you use the proper bar. Dove, Neutrogena, and PanOxyl are a few examples which are best bar cleaning soap choices for the face.

2. Make a decision if you need a medicated or non-medicated choice.

Medicated pimples cleansers are to be had each over-the-counter and with a prescription, and probably contain benzoyl peroxide, salicylic acid, or sulfur.

Standard use of a medicated cleanser can aid slash pore blockages and breakouts. Should you are not utilising another medication product, a medicated purifier is an efficient alternative.

If you're currently utilizing an extra pimples remedy remedy, like Retin-A or Accutane, a medicated cleaner will undoubtedly depart your skin too dry and uncomfortable.

 You'll want to pick a non-medicated purifier instead. Are trying some thing supposed for touchy dead   -- like Aveeno, Cetaphil, or Eucerin.

Three. Make certain the cleaner is meant on your face, and now not your body.

The skin for your face, neck and décolleté (chest area) is relatively thin and tender. So at the same time that tremendous smelling, extremely cleansing body wash is nice for in different places on the physique, it is not a just right choice for your face.

If a cleanser is meant for the body, it will have to simplest be used on the physique. More advantageous doesn't suggest better, specifically when it comes to your skin . Invariably use a cleaner that's certainly designed for the face, to cut back the threat of irritation.

4. Center of attention on the way it makes your skin suppose, now not on the price.

High-priced facial cleansers don't necessarily work any better than discount merchandise you can find at your nearby drug or reduction store. So don't fear if you can not find the money for a costly product (or just don't want to spend an arm and a leg!) You are not doing all of your skin a disservice by making a choice on a great purchase over today's packaging.

A greater guide is to move with how the cleaner makes your skin consider. Is your skin tight, dry, or itchy after you use it? It is now not the proper cleaner for you. Are trying an additional company.

5. Ask for a advice.

Still overwhelmed? Ask the professionals!

If you are seeing a dermatologist, ask him/her first. Not simplest will your doc have effective cleansers in intellect, however is aware of exactly which acne drugs you're using.

You'll be able to get personalized recommendations.

A further choice is an esthetician. Your esthetician can propose cleansers, and frequently could have them on sale so that you can take dwelling.

5 affordable Benzoyl Peroxide Cleansers for Treating pimples at dwelling

Benzoyl peroxide is by and large the primary over-the-counter healing option for people with acne, specially slight cases that can be treated with drugstore merchandise. Fortunately, you don't must spend so much for an amazing benzoyl peroxide purifier.

Most pimples therapies dry the skin to a point, so overuse of these merchandise would intent excessive dryness, peeling, and redness. You may wish to start with a single pimples therapy product, and slowly add extra if needed. That is certainly genuine if your skin tends to be touchy or readily irritated.

Part of the battle in treating acne   is finding merchandise that be just right for you. You may also must experiment with a couple of remedy merchandise before discovering one that improves your acne , so try not to get discouraged, and check out to be patient.

After several weeks of treating your pimples with over-the-counter products, when you aren't seeing growth, don't hesitate to contact your health care professional.

Here are some benzoyl peroxide cleansers you can also like that won't destroy the bank.

Smooth and Clear continuous control pimples cleaner

If you're looking for a common cleaner, this one by clean and Clear suits the bill. It contains 10 percent benzoyl peroxide, to help decrease the amount of acne -inflicting micro organism. Use in position of your typical purifier a few times per day.

This is a nice cleaner to aid cut down oily shine. It could possibly dry your skin , though, so make sure you employ an oil-free moisturizer daily.

Neutrogena Clear Pore cleaner / masks

Neutrogena has lengthy been a skin care staple. This purifier has a smooth odor and leaves the dead feeling cool and refreshed. And do not suppose that when you consider that it comprises less benzoyl peroxide than different choices (three.5%) that it's not robust.

PanOxyl 10% acne cleaning Bar

if you'd as an alternative have a cleansing bar, you may also like this one from PanOxyl. You should utilize it on your face, as good as the chest, again, shoulders, and other pimples-inclined areas.

But ensure to make use of this bar handiest on those acne-inclined areas: there isn't any experience in utilising it to cleanse your ft! Using this bar on areas without acne will simplest lead to needless drying of the skin.

With 10% benzoyl peroxide, it can be the absolute best force that you can get over the counter, making it an exceptionally good alternative for body breakouts. PanOxyl also offers a ten% acne

Foaming Wash and four% pimples Creamy Wash that you could be decide upon for facial cleansers.

Oxy every day Wash

The packaging recommendations advocate utilising two to 3 instances per day, but that could leave you feeling fairly dry and flaky. You could need to off making use of this product just as soon as per day, and slowly work up to twice daily in case your skin can manage it. You too can want to take a look at Oxy Face Wash sensitive, with 5 percentage benzoyl peroxide.

Neaclear Liquid Oxygen acne cleaner

This cleanser gives you the appear and think of an luxurious company, for a lot less. It does a first-class job of eliminating makeup, and it involves nutrients A, D, C, and E together with benzoyl peroxide.

Treating acne with Topical Erythromycin

it could be great if pimples would at all times be sorted with over-the-counter merchandise. However, as you may good have skilled, that is no longer at all times the case.

Most likely, to get some actual outcome you'll be able to have to turn to your doctor for a prescription acne treatment. The excellent news is, there are a lot of topical medicinal drugs which might be super robust in treating acne.

So, if OTC acne merchandise just are not helping, it is time to move on to the prescription options.

(not sure if you are able for a prescription acne treatment? This text: Do I desire a Prescription therapy? Will help you make a decision.)

Azelaic Acid

Azelaic acid is a prescription cream or gel for moderate to average acne .

It is believed that azelaic acid works by reducing Propionibacteria acnes, the micro organism accountable for acne breakouts. It also helps normalize shedding of dead skin cells, and decreases infection. Azelaic acid has the introduced advantage of improving post-inflammatory hyperpigmentation, the discoloration left after an pimples lesion has healed.

Azelaic acid can also be bought underneath the brand names Azelex and Finacea.

Topical Retinoids

Topical retinoids are tremendously trendy and mighty pimples remedies. Topical retinoids are a gaggle of medicines derived from synthetic nutrition A.

The topical retinoids which might be used to treat pimples include tretinoin and tazarotene. Adapalene is more adequately described as a retinoid-like compound, however considering it really works in simply the identical manner it can be probably incorporated in the topical retinoid team

Topical retinoids speedily exfoliate the skin , keeping your pores unclogged and preventing comedones. They may be used to deal with slight to moderate breakouts, as well as severe acne .

Topical retinoids, specifically the topical retinoid tretinoin, produce other advantages -- they are potent anti-aging cures.

They're most often used to diminish the look of first-rate lines and wrinkles, making retinoids a popular medication choice for adult onset pimples sufferers.

The most customary topical retinoids used to treat acne are:

• Differin (adapalene)

• Retin-A (tretinoin)

• Retin-A Micro (tretinoin)

• Avage (tazarotene)

• Tazorac (tazarotene)

Topical Antibiotics

Topical antibiotics reinforce acne by stopping the development of acne -inflicting micro organism, propioni acnes. They are able to also aid minimize inflammation and might diminish the amount of blocked pores.

Topical antibiotics don't seem to be used as in general at present as they had been in years past in view that they are able to contribute to antibiotic-resistant bacteria. To counteract this predicament, topical antibiotics will have to be used along with one more pimples cure treatment, like a topical retinoid or benzoyl peroxide.

Topical antibiotics are usually prescribed for average to severe acne . The most common topical antibiotics used to deal with acne are clindamycin and erythromycin.

Topical mixture medicines

Topical mixture medicinal drugs, as the name suggests, comprise drugs which contain two acne-fighting components.

You get the advantages of both medicinal drugs with just one software.

These medicinal drugs can kill pimples-inflicting bacteria, normalize the shedding of dead dead cells, keep pores clear, and diminish the quantity of comedones, depending on the combo acne medication that your dermatologist prescribes.

An predominant feature of topical combo therapy is the truth that less antibiotic is in general needed to kill bacteria in comparison with making use of topical antibiotics alone.

There are a lot of topical blend treatment choices, together with:

- Acanya (clindamycin and benzoyl peroxide)

- Benzamycin (benzoyl peroxide and erythromycin)

- BenzaClin (benzoyl peroxide and clindamycin)

- Duac (benzoyl peroxide and clindamycin)

- Epiduo (adapalene and benzoyl peroxide)

- Onexton (clindamycin and benzoyl peroxide)

- Ziana (clindamycin and tretinoin)

Your Dermatologist Can Prescribe the right medicine for You

there are such a large amount of prescription remedy choices to be had to treat acne . Fortunately, your dermatologist will recognize in order to work the nice on your breakouts.

Prescription medications can work rapidly. Inside only a few weeks, that you may begin noticing development of your skin. So, don't wait any longer. Provide your dermatologist a name.

You're typically familiar with antibiotics; odds are that you've got used them at some factor in your existence. They are used to deal with any style of bacterial contamination.

Considering that acne is, partially, brought about by means of micro organism, topical antibiotics (that means, you observe them to the dead) are one strategy to get pimples underneath manage. Oral antibiotics are used to deal with acne , too.

There are a lot of one-of-a-kind forms of antibiotics. The ones used most mainly to treat acne topically are clindamycin and erythromycin.

Topical tetracycline is in many instances used too, but much less in general when you consider that it has the tendency to show the skin yellow.

Topical antibiotics are used to deal with slight to moderately extreme inflammatory acne. They arrive in a sort of types, including lotions, gels, pads (pledgets) and toner-like solutions.

Here's How They Work

similar to oral antibiotics, topical antibiotics inhibit the development of micro organism. A major rationale of acne is the proliferation of the acne-inflicting bacteria Propionibacteria acnes, or P. Acnes.

This bacterium is an typical resident of the skin, but in those with acne the P. Acnes populace grows out of control. These bacteria irritate the dead 's follicles, growing infected papules and pustules.

Applying a topical antibiotic reduces the quantity of P. Acnes, which in flip helps control pimples. Topical antibiotics additionally diminish inflammation, so that they work best for inflamed breakouts as a substitute than non-infected blemishes or blackheads.

Topical Antibiotics aren't Used as the only real acne remedy

Topical antibiotics are not used on their own to treat acne, or as a minimum they more commonly just isn't.

Far more attention is paid to the very fact of antibiotic resistance. Utilising topical antibiotics by myself to deal with pimples can make contributions to this problem.

  Then you'll finish up with pimples that just is not going to reply to that type of antibiotic anymore.

Some medical professionals think that topical erythromycin is not as powerful because it was in treating pimples exactly due to the fact that of antibiotic resistant bacteria. Using a further acne medication along with your topical antibiotic can support restrict this hindrance from taking place.

Plus, topical antibiotics on my own simply don't seem to be the excellent technique to treat acne . They work really slowly when compared to different topical acne cures on hand. Who relatively desires to wait longer than they ought to before seeing results?

And even as they scale back bacteria and irritation, they do nothing to cut down pore blockages and the formation of microcomedones (the tiny beginnings of a pimple beneath the dead).

Other acne   remedies help Topical Antibiotics Work higher

regularly, your healthcare professional will also prescribe a different acne   cure to be used along with topical antibiotics. Benzoyl peroxide is a probable choice. It works well with topical antibiotics, and might support lessen the likelihood of developing antibiotic-resistant bacteria.

Topical retinoids are a further choice that work good with topical antibiotics. These quickly exfoliate your skin , decreasing the formation of comedones (blocked pores).

For grownup women with hormonal pimples, topical antibiotics might also be mixed with oral medications like spironolactone or beginning manipulate capsules.

Your dermatologist will recognize which medicinal drugs are the satisfactory match for you.

Prescription medicinal drugs That incorporate Topical Antibiotics

There are some acne   remedies to be had that mix both topical antibiotics with yet another treatment treatment. A few of these combo medicines are:

Benzamycin (erythromycin and benzoyl peroxide)

Acanya, BenzaClin, and Duac (clindamycin and benzoyl peroxide)

Ziana (clindamycin and tretinoin)

relying to your skin , any such possibly a excellent fit for you. Once more, your dermatologist will help create the first-rate medication plan.

Feasible side effects of Topical Antibiotics

The possible facet effects depend on the kind of remedy you're utilizing, but most men and women can use topical antibiotics readily. Aspect results, when they do happen, are not typically too bothersome.

You would get some dryness, flakiness, or minor peeling of the skin . Your treatment may burn or sting quite when it's utilized. Some topical antibiotic medications could reason some mild skin inflammation.

Serious facet results from topical antibiotics are very rare.

Even supposing topical antibiotics don't seem to be the correct choice for you, your dermatologist has plenty of therapy choices to support get your acne below control. So, do not wait any more. Make that appointment today!

Erythromycin is a topical antibiotic that's used to treat inflammatory acne . It comes in many differnt types, from lotions, gels, and ointments, to toner-like options and pledgets (small pads soaked in medicated resolution, just like a Stridex pad.)

you can most effective get topical erythromycin with a prescription. Oral erythromycin can also be used to deal with acne.

The way it Works

One element of acne development is a proliferation of acne-causing micro organism within the pore.

The propionibacterium acnes is the manager culprit here. Antibiotics like erythromycin cut back the quantity of acne - inflicting micro organism and contamination.

Topical erythromycin may also support scale back redness and inflammation.

Topical Erythromycin isn't the first healing choice

Topical erythromycin itself is not the first remedy choice for acne . It isn't tremendously robust towards acne, and there are a lot of different choices that effortlessly work higher.

Topical erythromycin only objectives one pimples-inflicting element: bacteria. There are other causes which are liable for acne breakouts, like irregular shedding of dead cells and the development of pore blockages, that topical erythromycin just would not handle.

More importantly, a big hindrance with topical antibiotics and erythromycin in specific, is antibiotic resistance. The bacterium that causes pimples has emerge as used to the medication, so it now not works in opposition to it.

In some cases, although, erythromycin is the satisfactory cure choice. For pregnant and breastfeeding moms, for illustration. It is usually prescribed to treat newborn child acne and childish pimples, if want be.

Getting the great results from Topical Erythromycin

if your dermatologist decides that topical erythromycin is needed to deal with your acne , there are some steps that may be taken to support get the pleasant viable outcome.

First, don't use erythromycin as the only acne treatment. It works significantly better if it's paired with a second pimples remedy, like benzoyl peroxide or a topical retinoid.

Benzamycin is an pimples therapy remedy that mixes topical erythromycin with benzoyl peroxide. This helps streamline your cure movements, providing you with the advantage of two pimples-combating elements in a single.

Secondly, to aid fight bacterial resistance you ideally will handiest use topical erythromycin for a short while. Once irritation is elevated, you could stop making use of the erythromycin. Hold using your second acne Remedy, though, to continue improving breakouts and preserve your pimples under control.

Feasible facet results of Topical Erythromycin

Most folks can use topical erythromycin with none issues in any respect. In the event you do improve part results, they're much like other acne cures: mild irritation, burning or stinging, redness, and dry dead . If facet results are bothering you, or for those who develop a rash, let your dermatologist be aware of.

One challenge of topical erythromycin medication is that it may possibly stop working over time. Again, blame bacterial resistance. Let your derm comprehend if it isn't working for you, or if acne comes back after clearing up.

Oral erythromycin is an antibiotic used to deal with reasonable to extreme inflammatory pimples, or pimples that isn't getting better with different cures. Erythromycin is also used topically to treat acne.

Apart from pimples, erythromycin is used to treat a vast kind of stipulations, from ear infections to rosacea. It's a prescription treatment and there is not any over-the-counter alternative.

How it Works

Erythromycin works to strengthen acne through reducing the quantity of pimples-causing micro organism, known as propionibacteria acnes, on the skin.

  It additionally lessens infection and redness that's caused by way of breakouts.

Oral erythromycin is just not fairly supposed for use as a long-term pimples healing. Ideally, you'll be able to take it for just a few months or simply except your acne starts to get better. Then you'll be able to stop using the erythromycin and continue acne medication with a different medication that is higher ideal to long-term use, like a topical mixture pimples treatment, oral contraceptives (for females), etc. Suppose of oral erythromycin as a soar start to get infection beneath manipulate.

Erythromycin isn't the primary Antibiotic alternative for acne

Erythromycin has been used for years to treat acne, even though newer antibiotics are the more fashionable alternative at present. It conveniently isn't probably the most powerful antibiotic medication for acne .

Probably the most other oral antibiotics that are used more probably to treat pimples are:

• Tetracycline

• Azithromycin

• Doxycycline

• Minocycline

• Clindamycin

Erythromycin continues to be the high-quality antibiotic alternative for pregnant or breastfeeding moms, though. It additionally can be used with the aid of more youthful youngsters for the reason that, not like one of the crucial different oral antibiotics, it won't cause tooth discoloration.

Antibiotic Resistance and Oral Erythromycin

You've quite often heard concerning the developing hindrance of bacterial resistance brought about by the overuse of antibiotics.

On account that of this, some individuals to find their acne doesn't respond good to erythromycin medication.

To aid combat antibiotic resistance, oral erythromycin shouldn't be the one cure you are using to clear your acne. It's going to work high-quality if it's mixed with a different acne healing treatment.

Topical retinoids and benzoyl peroxide work rather well when used alongside oral antibiotics.

Feasible part effects of Oral Erythromycin

All acne drugs have them, and oral erythromycin is no distinct. Your dermatologist will let you know all about possible facet effects before you begin your healing, however these are probably the most customary:

• Upset stomach

• Nausea and vomiting

• Diarrhea

• Vaginal yeast infections or oral thrush

when you boost severe stomach agony or extreme diarrhea, let your doctor be aware of proper away. Is erythromycin upsetting your belly? Taking your erythromycin with meals can help.

Oral antibiotics work excellent when there's a constant amount of the treatment within the physique. Do your nice to take your medicine at typical times and try to not pass doses.

Make sure you take the entire course prescribed, even though your pimples clears up. Tell your dermatologist in case your pimples isn't improving at all, or if it will get better for a whilst however then returns.

Answers to the 5 Most normal questions about cleaning Your acne -prone dead

Are bar soaps ok?

Distinctive bar soaps can be utilized for cleansing the face. Dove and Neutrogena are two examples of bar soaps which are soft and suitable to make use of for cleaning your face.

What you need to prevent are antibacterial, deodorant physique bars. Whilst they work well for cleansing tougher areas like your back or toes, these soap bars could also be drying for the face.

Extra most important is the pH of the cleaning soap. Cleansers with an extraordinarily excessive pH (very alkaline) are going to be very drying and most likely stressful to the skin.

Typically, you will have to prefer a cleaner especially formulated for use on the face. These varieties of cleansers will provide you with a gentler cleaning than a bar of soap intended for use on the body in the bathe.

Should i take advantage of a washcloth or scrubbing pads?

These objects don't seem to be wanted to get a excellent, thorough cleansing of the skin. It will look that a excellent scrubbing would aid cleanse out the pores, but you probably have inflammatory acne scrubbing away at the skin can additional inflammation.

As an alternative, use just the pads of your fingers, therapeutic massage your cleanser over the face absolutely, and rinse very good.

In case your face feels exceptionally oily, or if you wear makeup, you are able to do a "double cleanse:" lather up, rinse, then repeat. Which you could additionally depart the cleaner on longer earlier than washing it off.

In the event you simply have got to use a washcloth or cleansing pad, select one that's soft and non-abrasive.

What temperature water should i exploit?

Room temperature water or simply hotter is the exceptional temperature to cleanse the face.

Many people swear with the aid of the "steaming hot water to open pores, icy cold to shut them" cleaning events. But this is not critical and may just sincerely be damaging to the skin . Water that's too scorching can contribute to couperose (broken capillaries), and exacerbate inflammation.

And bloodless water isn't needed to "shut" pores. Pores don't seem to be like doorways; they do not open and shut. You cannot alternate pore measurement with water.

If significant pores are a problem, are trying an alpha hydroxy acid (AHA) product. AHAs cast off dead skin cells and hardened oil plugs, making pores show up smaller. Gentle chemical peels, microdermabrasion, and retinoids might also make the pores seem smaller.

How typically will have to I cleanse my face?

How commonly should I cleanse my face?

Cleaning too by and large is not going to support the skin. The skin wants some normal oil to be healthy (yes, oil is usually a excellent thing). Cleansing too by and large can strip the skin of its natural oil, leading to over-dryness and inflammation.

On the whole, a twice-every day cleansing is enough to eliminate dust, excess oil, and make-up without stripping the skin. If you happen to've been exercising, are sweaty or notably dirty (like, after working within the yard) which you could throw one more cleanse in there for excellent measure.

And be certain you at all times wash your face earlier than mattress to cleanse away the filth and oil from the day and leave your skin ready for those topical pimples medicines.

Do Pore Strips Work?

Watching as an alternative like an oddly-formed Band-support, with tremendous sticky adhesive on one side, pore strips are pressed firmly onto the skin anywhere you have blackheads. The strip sets for a number of minutes, and then is pulled off of the skin .

The proposal is the adhesive will keep on with the top of your blackheads and pull them out of the pore.

Do Pore Strips rather Work? Yes and No

Pore strips give a quick, albeit temporary, growth of blackheads.

So in that appreciate, pore strips do work. But for a long run fix for blackheads, pore strips are not the first-rate option to go.

Pore Strips Can beef up the seem of Blackheads

as soon as you've gotten yanked the strip off of your face, go forward and take a look at what's been captured by way of the glue. You'll be able to see a veritable forest of little blackheads sticking straight up off the strip.

Your skin , too, will seem less congested. It will commonly additionally seem crimson. The strips do pull on the dead pretty aggressively. Luckily the redness subsides particularly swiftly.

To get the first-class viable outcome, you have got to use the pore strips exactly as directed. The guidelines differ reasonably from manufacturer to manufacturer, so make certain you read the guidelines for your product.

Pore strips can irritate the dead , so maintain that in intellect. You do not want to use them too most often. When you've obtained certainly sensitive dead , it can be most commonly high-quality to stay away altogether.

Pore Strips can not stop Blackheads from Forming

have you ever ever squeezed a blackhead? Then you know how long that plug of gunk is.

Pore strips pull off the highest, most seen part of the blackhead. Even as the tops of blackheads fill your pore strip, the relaxation of the blemish stays in the back of in the pore.

Despite the fact that blackheads seem fairly stable, they simply have more of a toothpaste-like consistency.

So the pore strips can not particularly clutch hold completely of anything semi-strong.

It's like hanging a piece of duct tape across the open tube of your toothpaste and ripping it off. Certain, there can be some toothpaste on the tape, however the majority will keep firmly encompassed in the tube. So does the blackhead to your pore.

Pore strips are not able to utterly take away higher, deeper blackheads. And, unluckily, they won't stop your blackheads from forming.

And here's a cool factoid for you -- did you know no longer all black dots on your nose are simply blackheads? It might be follicular prominence. They appear like tiny blackheads, but it's clearly tremendous, or prominent, pores. Pore strips will not support this in any respect.

No matter how almost always you use pore strips, they're by no means going to do away with your blackheads fully. For that, you will want a different cure. Learn on!

Use Pore Strips as a device, not Your foremost Blackhead remedy

in case you've most effective acquired a few blackheads right here and there, an occasional pore strip will commonly work simply quality for you.

But if blackheads are a primarily cussed hindrance, or you've got extra than just the occasional breakout, you are going to need whatever more powerful than a pore strip.

First, are trying an over-the-counter acne cure. The most mighty ones will include salicylic acid.

You would even decide to make an appointment at your neighborhood salon or skin spa. An esthetician can manually clean out blackheads and pore blockages, developing an immediate improvement of the skin. Like pore strips, extractions don't hold blackheads from forming, but can be a good bounce- to blackhead cure.

You probably have quite a lot of blackheads, and also you can not get growth with OTC pimples merchandise, it is time for a prescription treatment. (significantly, see a dermatologist for blackheads? Most likely!) Your derm will more commonly prescribe a topical retinoid to help get these blackheads beneath manipulate.

Is It Ever okay to Pop a Pimple or Squeeze a Blackhead?

How one can safely pop a pimple and extract a blackhead

we all know, we all know – don't pop acne . But who among us hasn't resorted to squeezing a blemish every once in a while?

No one wants to stroll around with a significant whitehead (or an apparent blackhead) on their face. What are you able to do in case you have a blemish that's simply begging to be sorted?

Is Popping a Pimple Ever good enough?

The absolute most secure factor to your skin is to keep a fingers-off procedure – letting the pimple heal naturally, without squeezing it.

When you squeeze a pimple, even though you may get some pus to drain, which you could even be forcing that contaminated material deeper into the pore. The stress can rationale the wall of the pore to burst beneath the outside of your skin .

This gunk now spreads to different pores and may purpose a brand new pimple to form. You additionally up your probabilities that the pimple will go away a everlasting scar.

That stated, it's tough to recreation a gigantic whitehead at work or institution. In this case, you can be competent to softly categorical the pus and allow the pimple to drain.

Before Resorting to Popping, try These methods

Popping isn't the one strategy to get that pimple to empty, although. Before resorting to popping, try these tricks first.

Have a reputable drain it for you: The great thing you can do is have a dermatologist or an esthetician drain the pimple or blackhead for you. The pros recognize tips on how to cautiously extract these blemishes with out causing harm to the skin.

Extractions work notably good for blackheads, and your therapist can do away with most of the blackheads for your skin in only one or two visits.

Of direction, we do not continuously have the time (or the cash) to run to the salon whenever a blemish appears. So, should you are not able to have the professionals do it, learn on.

Are trying a warm compress: if in case you have a pustule with a massive, apparent white head, that you could attempt to get it to drain with a warm compress.

Simply soak a gentle material in warm water and preserve it over the pimple for a few minutes. Rewarm the compress when it will get bloodless.

The warmness helps to soften the top and permits the pimple to drain naturally. Ensure, though, that the pustule is "competent," with a giant white head on the floor of the skin. When you do that with a pimple before the white head has fashioned, that you could virtually make the blemish appear bigger and more infected.

Additionally, this approach is not going to work on blackheads.

Spot treat it: when you have a day or with the intention to wait, spot cures are yet another good approach to dry up that whitehead. Just dab a small amount on the pimple and go away it alone. In most cases the spot remedy will dry up that pimple overnight.

Which you can get spot therapies over-the-counter, in the skin care aisle of your neighborhood drug store. Products that incorporate benzoyl peroxide or sulfur tend to work high-quality on pustules. Some folks even have excellent results with merchandise containing salicylic acid or tea tree oil. You may also need to test with a number of different brands to find the one that works pleasant for your skin .

If you have to, this is tips on how to Safely Pop a Pimple

Ideally, you'll be in a position to take care of your pimple without squeezing. Popping acne should perpetually be a final resort.

Should you suppose like you must pop that whitehead, although, i might as an alternative you do it safely. Don't forget, at any time when you squeeze a blemish there's no assurance that you will not harm your skin . However these steps will as a minimum lessen that hazard.

This handiest works for blemishes with colossal, obvious white heads which can be almost the outside of the dead .

Step 1: Wash your fingers good with soap and water.

Step 2: Sanitize a needle or pin with rubbing alcohol.

Step three: Coming parallel to the dead , gently prick the highest of the whitehead with the tip of the needle. Don't go so deep that you simply draw blood! You simply want to pierce the very floor of the whitehead.

Step 4: Wrap your fingers in tissue or cotton. Situation your fingers on both side of the blemish. Instead of compacting, though, gently pull faraway from the blemish. This on the whole drains the pimple without you having to squeeze at all, lowering the chances of pushing contaminated fabric deeper into the skin.

If this works, congrats, that you would be able to discontinue right here! No have got to squeeze in any respect.

Step 5: still have the whitehead? Clutch two cotton swabs, and follow smooth stress to the sides of the blemish. This can be a gentler system than using your fingers.

Don't squeeze to the factor of drawing blood – simply ample to drain the whitehead. Observe a tiny dab of antibacterial ointment to the pimple.

If the pimple would not drain readily, it can be not ready. Do not drive it. It can be exceptional to leave it on my own. Are trying an overnight spot healing in the intervening time.

Never, Ever try to Pop a Deep, inflamed Blemish

at the same time you could normally gently extract a whitehead, there are designated types of acne   you will have to on no account attempt to pop.

Any pink pimple with no white head (papules) must certainly not be squeezed. These significant, inflamed, deep blemishes (nodular breakouts and cysts) should in no way be squeezed either.

Is your blemish certainly huge and really painful? You'll be able to need to go away this blemish on my own, too. It may not be a pimple in any respect, but as a substitute a boil.

The way to Safely Extract a Blackhead

it is frequently safer to extract a blackhead than an inflamed pimple. There may be less danger of infection and scarring.

Nonetheless, this isn't license to digging away at your skin . You'll be able to still ought to deal with your skin gently.

Step 1: Wash your arms with cleaning soap.

Step 2: Wrap your fingers in cotton or tissue. Location tender pressure on both facet of the blackhead. Attempt to get down underneath the blackhead and push up cautiously.

Instead of regular pressure, use extra of rocking or massaging motion to support loosen the plug. Continue this until the core is completely extracted. Don't forget, do not practice so much stress that you just draw blood!

Comedo extractors, those small steel tools estheticians use to eliminate blackheads, are a different alternative. But be conscious, these can do extra damage than excellent in unskilled palms. That you could with ease follow too much stress and bruise your skin .

When you do use a comedo extractor, ensure you sanitize it first with rubbing alcohol. Position the loop of the extractor across the blackhead. Put gentle pressure straight down; do not use the extractor to dig on the blackhead. If you are leaving crimson marks on the skin , you are pushing too difficult.

Some blackheads are cussed and do not want to depart the pore. When you cannot extract them, depart them on my own for an extra day.

Step 3: Use a toner or astringent on the entire areas that you have extracted.

Obtained various Blemishes?

Use an acne healing to stop breakouts before they start.

Extracting individual blemishes on occasion is not a colossal deal. But when you have tons of breakouts, the satisfactory choice is to stop them earlier than they even show up. For that, you'll want an acne   healing that you can use day-to-day.

Over-the-counter acne products will also be beneficial for blackheads and moderate acne . If OTC therapies aren't doing the trick, there are a lot of prescription pimples medicinal drugs so that it will work on each inflammatory acne and blackheads.

If you want help getting your blemishes below manipulate, make an appointment with a dermatologist.

6 approaches To Heal a Pimple that you've Picked, Popped or Squeezed

You had a pimple that was once using you loopy. So you popped it (yeah, you already know you shouldn't pop acne but oftentimes you simply can't support your self). Now, alternatively of a pimple, you have an indignant purple sore or a dry crusty scab.

Here are some guidelines for the way to hinder that former pimple (now nasty scab) from getting worse.

Do not prefer at acne

First matters first, you have to enable the popped pimple to heal.

That means no more messing with it. Don't squeeze it to peer if any longer will come out. Don't decide upon on the scab. Let your skin the therapy method with out being interrupted.

Hold the skin clean

when you've simply popped a pimple, go ahead and give it a excellent cleaning. You need to use your general facial cleaner for this as you're washing your face. Be smooth, though, and check out to not knock off the scab that is trying to kind.

You could additionally use a touch of witch hazel on a cotton ball or swab. Carefully dab the popped pimple with this solution a couple of times a day, as a minimum except a just right scab forms.

Even though plenty of persons advocate cleansing a popped pimple with rubbing alcohol or hydrogen peroxide, those can sting, and don't seem to be as potent as witch hazel as decreasing any irritation that will arise.

Practice Ice to a Former Pimple

when you have a colossal, inflamed, pink bump in your face, ice is the pleasant method to soothe it.

Use an ice cube or bloodless %, both wrapped in a soft material or paper towel and ice it down. This may increasingly support cut down the swelling and make your popped pimple consider better.

In case your popped pimple already has a scab, and it's no longer swollen in any respect, icing the field is not going to do some thing so just bypass this step.

Treat Popped acne with Antibiotic Ointment

deal with your popped pimple like an open wound, given that that is in actual fact what it's.

Over-the-counter antibiotic ointment is your great buddy. Dot a small quantity straight on the popped pimple or scab. This will help pace up cure time. It also maintains the scab moist, so it is not going to seem as dry, crackly, and apparent.

Preserve a picked-at pimple included with a small quantity of ointment except it's thoroughly healed. This can take a couple of days.

Also, be certain you are best masking the pimple, now not the skin around it (above all if it's in your face). Non-prescription antibiotic ointment may clog your pores, so you wish to have to maintain it simply within the field where it is needed.

Don't pick at a Scabbed Pimple

it can be tempting, but do not provide in. You want that scab to stay put to your pimple to heal. If you're a bona fide picker, do your first-rate to maintain your palms off of your face. Again, retaining the scab blanketed with remedy ointment makes it less appealing to decide upon it off.

Proceed utilising pimples treatments.

If you're utilizing any OTC acne products or prescription acne medications, you should continue to do so. Most acne drugs have antibacterial homes which must be priceless in getting that pimple to heal.

Keep in mind, for those who deal with your popped pimple well, it will have to heal within a number of days. You need to be sufferer except this happens.

acne remedy hints for the Bride and Groom

Congratulations in your engagement!

You want your wedding day to be excellent, from the plant life and music to your dress or tux. However if in case you have pimples you will have another significant worry -- how your skin will seem on the marriage ceremony day.

Despite the fact that nothing can assurance flawless dead in your marriage ceremony, the proper administration can extensively improve acne. Comply with these steps to aid get your acne under manipulate earlier than your marriage ceremony.

As far upfront as feasible:

See a healthcare professional and devise a therapy plan. You would spend months jumping from one over-the-counter treatment to one other with obviously no improvement in any respect. When you are on a closing date it's first-class to deliver within the professionals correct away.

Acne treatments do not work in a single day, and you may also have got to are trying a few choices earlier than hitting on one who works for you. Keep time in your part. See a healthcare professional as soon as viable to ensure treatments have a lot of time to work.

Even if you don't want a prescription pimples therapy, your dermatologist can advocate robust OTC merchandise, saving you money and time looking round.

Speak about the chances for scar remedy. Your dermatologist can even support you if acne scar therapies are wanted. More often than not, your health practitioner will need acne to be beneath manage before beginning a scar healing software.

Even though you do not need proper scarring, many people to find that as their pimples begins to clear they're left with uneven skin tone, or submit-inflammatory hyperpigmentation.

Your derm has treatments that may improve this too. Again, enable for a lot of time for these treatments to work.

10-365 days earlier than:

start a strict skin care regimen. A good skin care events will incorporate cleansing, exfoliating, moisturizing and solar protection, and will include your pimples treatment medicines.

Head to your nearest day spa. You may wish to spend money on a series of pimples therapy facials. A good-informed esthetician may give deep-cleaning facial treatments and extract cussed blackheads. She'll also endorse skin care products if you're feeling overwhelmed via alternatives.

Consider, though, that an esthetician isn't a substitute for a dermatologist. There are matters an esthetician cannot do for pimples.

If you are using prescription acne medicinal drugs, get your doctor's ok earlier than having a facial completed. Also tell the esthetician about any acne medication you're utilizing, even over-the-counter merchandise.

Eight-10 Months before:

guide a makeup artist. If you're opting to have a professional do your make-up, now's the time to start lining one up. Meet with a few makeup artists, and let them show you their work.

A excellent make-up artist can aid camouflage breakouts, so even if your skin is not rather superb by the time your marriage ceremony arrives, as a minimum it might seem love it is. The exceptional makeup artists are busy, so guide your date well in advance.

Grooms -- ask your bride-to-be's make-up artist to carve out a couple of minutes to contact up any blemishes you've gotten. Don't worry, this is a normal practice and the outcome are very normal.

There are numerous pimples cover up options for guys. Many makeup artists offer this carrier as a part of a bundle.

6-8 Months earlier than:

Take stock of what is working, and what is not. Let your health practitioner know how the remedies are working. Are you noticing facet results? Are you seeing improvement? There is still time to take a look at one other cure if needed.

Generally, acne treatments do not work well no longer due to the fact they are not effective, but because they aren't getting used safely. Make certain you realize exactly tips on how to use your remedy, and follow these guidelines exactly. Ask your health care professional if you are uncertain.

4-6 Months before:

manipulate stress. By using now you are completely immersed in wedding-planning small print and commencing to suppose the pressure. A couple of experiences have shown a hyperlink between acne severity and stress. There is a lot of anecdotal evidence as well.

Take a lot of time to de-stress. Try yoga, meditation, reading, running, or every other recreation that helps you believe more centered. If alleviating stress doesn't help your skin, it'll at least aid you enjoy the marriage ceremony planning.

2-four Months before:

continue utilising your therapies always. You're busy planning all those last-minute important points, but don't let your acne therapies fall by using the wayside. Recall, consistency is essential, so no skipping days! (listed below are some pointers to aid you don't forget your treatments, even to your busiest days.)

additionally, do not let your busy time table preempt your dermatologist visits. Retaining them now's just as ESSENCIAL as ever.

Even supposing your skin is clear, keep utilising your medications diligently. Acne therapies do not therapy acne ; they simply manipulate it. When you discontinue making use of them pimples is more likely to return.

1-2 Months before:

schedule your final facial remedy. If you've been having regular facials, get your last medication executed a few weeks prior to the marriage ceremony.

Don't get a facial less than one week before the marriage ceremony, above all a process like microdermabrasion, chemical peels, and even extractions. The final thing you wish to have is a red or splotchy complexion for the wedding.

If you're eager on having a salon remedy carried out, as a substitute of a facial are attempting a calming therapeutic massage or body wrap rather.

1-2 Weeks before:

don't are attempting any new cures. Now just isn't the time to begin a brand new acne medication or skin care product. The last thing you need is a response to a brand new product, or excessively dry, peeling skin.

Do not opt for, pop, or squeeze. With the wedding simply across the nook, you are opening to scrutinize your skin . Face up to the urge to pop these pimples.

Selecting at the blemishes can set off more irritation and only makes acne appear worse. Plus, makeup can quilt a blemish extra easily than it will probably a scab. So don't pop!

Oops! Already made that mistake? This is how you can heal a picked at pimple quick.

1-2 Days earlier than:

Get a cortisone shot. It is every body's worst worry -- a colossal pimple showing just before the wedding day.

Cortisone injections to the rescue! A cortisone shot helps reduce inflammation and flattens out these enormous blemishes, repeatedly inside a subject just a few hours.

Talk to your physician concerning the possibility of having a cortisone shot executed earlier than you desperately want one. Then, if the necessity arises which you could be inside and outside, with out a tremendous fuss.

Day of the marriage ceremony:

calm down! If your skin is not as clear as you would like, don't panic. Recollect, makeup can do wondrous matters. Let the make-up artists do their work.

If you're doing all of your possess make-up, use a dab of green concealer to duvet pink blemishes. Cover with dead -toned concealer and a dusting of powder. (you'll be able to wish to apply and ultimate this system before your wedding day.) Grooms -- ask a sister, cousin, or female buddy for support.

Revel in your marriage ceremony day! Bear in mind, your skin issues are extra seen to you than they are to someone else. Do not agonize over acne , just enjoy your wedding. Finally the training, you deserve it.

The right way to Shave The right means you probably have pimples

Shaving when you've got acne generally is a bit complex. If you're now not cautious shaving round acne, it can be effortless to be left with uncooked, crimson, burning skin.

In need of tossing your razor and developing a beard that may make ZZ prime green with envy, what can you do?

Even though it takes only a bit extra care, that you would be able to stay moderately smooth-shaven and nonetheless treat your skin gently, whilst allowing acne to heal.

Don't Shave Over acne

First and main, don't attempt to difficult it out and shave correct over the pimples.

Significantly — ouch! That's undoubtedly now not excellent for your skin .

Shaving the tops off of pimples gained't aid them clear rapid. What it may do is open your skin up to infection and possible scarring.

It also prolongs the medication approach, turning that pimple into an open sore and then a scab that takes much longer to depart. Not to point out, acne remedies can sting relatively a little bit when utilized to broken dead .

As an alternative of shaving over pimples, try to shave round inflamed blemishes as so much as possible.

Swap to an electrical Razor or Single Blade

those fairly excellent multi-blade razors supply a great close shave. They also create numerous friction and drag when it is pulled across the dead . That, my buddies, will also be enormously anxious to already inflamed damaged-out skin .

If your acne looks and feels worse after shaving together with your multi-blade razor, try switching to a best quality single blade razor or an electric razor instead.

You will not get as delicate a shave, however these razors are so much less stressful and gentler on already inflamed skin.

Ditch the Shave and Trim rather

For some guys, shaving itself can set off a breakout. If even careful shaving causes considerable redness and inflammation, you may want to ditch the razor altogether.

Alternatively, use a trimmer to keep your self good-groomed.

Considering that a trimmer isn't dragging across the skin, you will not get that friction burn you get with a razor. It will not be an ultimate approach to shave but it surely is the most gentle. And if your breakouts are particularly standard, it might not be sensible to shave round each and every pimple anyway.

You can use this system best in the midst of a bad breakout, or change to it full-time, depending on how sensitive your skin is and how severe your acne.

Make particular it is really pimples

There are other skin conditions that rationale acne -like bumps and acne, especially in the beard subject.

Very long-established is a called pseudofolliculitis barbae. We all know this by the extra customary time period "razor bumps." The purpose of that is, sarcastically, shaving itself.

When the hair is shaved close, it might probably intent the hair to develop into the skin alternatively than up out of the pore because it in general does. These ingrown hairs can seem rather like acne , and can regularly be fallacious for acne.

Suspect pseudofolliculitis barbae if the pimples only occur in the bear area. Your health care professional can support you diagnose the hindrance if you are unsure.

Start an pimples cure movements to Banish Breakouts for just right

The ideal drawback is one where acne is long past, making the above tips moot. Your acne can be cleared up. You just must find the right therapy.

If your pimples is mild, which you could with over-the-counter pimples treatments first. (no longer certain? Listed here are indicators you're coping with mild acne .)

try the over-the-counter acne product for a number of weeks. In the event you get excellent outcome, maintain using it! Stopping use of acne remedies permits acne to come, so plan on utilising your pimples treatments for the lengthy haul.

If OTC merchandise simply aren't chopping it, make a shuttle to the dermatologist. There are plenty of prescription pimples drugs that can begin clearing breakouts as a substitute quickly, inside a few weeks. So, give your dermatologist a name.

Some thing medication you prefer, perpetually treat your skin gently. Let it heal. Even as shaving take your time, are trying now not to rush, and be careful with your skin .

Why OTC acne products do not Work:

3 rapid Fixes for Getting results from Over-the-Counter acne merchandise

you have acne . You head to the drugstore and purchase an acne therapy purifier. You use mentioned purifier for a few weeks. You continue to have acne . So, you head to the drugstore and buy an acne treatment toner. Use it; nonetheless have acne. Repeat for months.

Sound familiar? It definite does for me. I did this dance for a long, long time earlier than i noticed that I was once doing a number of things mistaken.

Listed here are 3 causes why over-the-counter acne cures aren't working – and what you are able to do to ensure you get specific results.

1

purpose#1: Your Product would not contain a verified acne therapy Ingredient

This doesn't appear really fair, however there aren't any principles in the market saying an over-the-counter pimples remedy product ought to include components that honestly tested to treat acne .

Many effectiveness of many ingredients determined in OTC merchandise haven't been totally studied. And when experiences were carried out, they are almost always completed by means of the manufacturers themselves. Makes you wonder in regards to the objectivity. Simply sayin'.

Fast fix: Get a product that involves proven acne healing ingredients.

Subsequent time you purchase an OTC acne product, assess out the energetic constituents. They are going to be listed on the bottle or box.

Look for salicylic acid, benzoyl peroxide, glycolic acid, or higher yet a mixture of these. (good enough, so glycolic acid isn't an pimples remedy per se, but it can help boost the effectiveness of alternative pimples cure materials.) These had been studied and verified amazing against acne .

Picking an OTC acne cure product can also be overwhelming, so I've put collectively a cheat-sheet with a view to support you when you head to the dead care aisle: how you can prefer an Over-the-Counter acne healing.

2

cause #2: You're utilizing just one healing Product

I'm going to assist you to in on a little secret – hanging together a couple of over-the-counter acne merchandise can give you significantly better outcome than just one.

There's a rationale why Proactiv, AcneFree, and other OTC acne cure leaders give you a package complete with cleaner, toner, mask, and lotion.

Acne is brought on by means of a couple of factors. Utilizing one-of-a-kind products with different lively ingredients gives pimples a one-two punch. You'll be focusing on quite a lot of breakout-causing factors at once and seeing the results seeing that of it.

Fast repair: Put together a complete acne medication activities with a few OTC pimples merchandise.

That you can buy all-inclusive pimples cure kits, or put collectively your own a-la-carte with products off the shelf. Right here's how: Create Your own OTC acne cure routine.

3

intent #three: Your pimples is too extreme to Be dealt with via OTC products

You might be doing the whole lot correct, and nonetheless no longer get just right outcome from over-the-counter acne merchandise. It's not your fault. It's going to with no trouble be you're no longer a excellent candidate for over-the-counter treatment.

OTC acne merchandise work excellent on mild pimples. If your pimples is moderate to extreme, deep or very infected, it's highly unlikely it's going to reply to the merchandise which you could buy on the drugstore.

But you're not out of good fortune! Despite the fact that OTC pimples merchandise aren't working, there are a lot of extra robust prescription choices with the intention to.

Rapid repair: Forgo over-the-counter acne cures and get a prescription remedy rather.

Adequate, so this isn't always a quick repair. It does imply a trip to see your doctor, which isn't almost as effortless as hitting the nook drugstore. However lengthy-time period, you're going to get more bang for your buck with a prescription acne   medicine.

You'll be so much happier with the outcome when you consider that which you can genuinely start getting improvement to your skin . Doesn't that make the commute to the dermatologist appear helpful?

So, should you're equipped, these articles will support you get started:

Why acne Come again while you stop utilising acne medicine

You used your pimples medication for weeks (or months) without fail. And also you were rewarded with clearer skin! You have been super pleased to eventually put those acne treatments on the shelf and overlook about them.

However as soon as you stopped using your acne medication, the acne came back. Did the remedy not work properly? Is your acne treatment just not mighty?

Why do the acne come back whilst you discontinue utilising your acne remedy?

Acne drugs do not therapy acne , they simply manage It

Most individuals anxiously look ahead to the day they'll not need to use their acne medications. Unfortunately, stopping remedy usually approach a return of pimples.

This does not imply that your medicine is not working. Actually, should you've had significant clearing, your medicinal drugs are genuinely working rather well.

Acne healing medicines do not therapy acne, and they don't discontinue the factors that intent acne within the first location. Alternatively, they simply manipulate these reasons to keep breakouts at bay.

Pimples is prompted, most commonly, by an overabundance of oil, dead dead cells, and acne -inflicting bacteria within the pore.

Pimples cure medications work through decreasing oil and micro organism, and help maintain pores cleared of dead skin cells.

But acne medicines do not change the best way your skin behaves. If healing is stopped, the pores grow to be impacted once more and breakouts return.

You can need to continue to make use of Your drugs Even After Your skin is apparent

To keep pimples from coming back, you'll be able to have got to hold making use of your acne medicines even after your skin is clear.

The awesome exception to this is isotretinoin. This medicine is the closest factor we ought to an precise pimples "medication." you can most effective use isotretinoin for a specified amount of time.

Most people handiest want one or two guides of treatment with this medication. Once acne is gone, it's most of the time gone for good.

All different acne cure drugs, whether over-the-counter or prescription, will must be used continually to preserve pimples from coming back. This means you can be making use of your benzoyl peroxide, topical retinoids, topical antibiotics (or anything cure you are presently making use of) over clear skin. This is what will maintain your skin clear.

As soon as your pimples is significantly cleared, though, you will be capable to scale down in your therapies. For illustration, instead of applying your salicylic acid twice daily you'll be able to lessen to a as soon as-a-day software. Or you may drop your oral antibiotics and proceed using Retin-A Micro alone.

Need support Devising a long-time period remedy Plan? Ask Your Dermatologist

so to maintain pimples clear, you are going to want a long-time period remedy plan.

If your acne is moderate, and you've got gotten excellent outcome with over-the-counter acne treatment merchandise, then you definitely will have to continue to use these merchandise as part of your every day skin care routine.

If you've been utilizing prescription pimples drugs, your dermatologist will aid map out a medication plan in order to help keep your rough-gained results. Don't change how you use your prescription medications without first speakme with your dermatologist.

Post-Inflammatory Hyperpigmentation : Is it a real pimples Scar?

Your acne is clearing up and your skin is watching higher every day. But then you definitely detect dark discolorations in all places the acne lesions have healed. Is it acne scarring?

Those dark spots are known as put up-inflammatory hyperpigmentation (frequently abbreviated PIH). It can be the medical term given to discoloration of the dead that follows an inflammatory wound.

Put up-inflammatory hyperpigmentation appears like flat areas of dark discolorations on the skin .

It will possibly happen at any place on the face and physique.

They can variety in color depending to your skin tone and depth of the discoloration. If you're fair-complected, your post-inflammatory hyperpigmentation spots are regularly going to be crimson to red, or crimson colored. Darker complexions will detect PIH spots are brown to black.

PIH spots is usually a variety of colors, however, the skin might not be pitted or depressed. It appears more like a discolored freckle on the skin , or perhaps a bigger, splotchy discoloration of the skin . Early on, these spots may appear brilliant, or like "new dead ."

Why do acne depart these discolored spots?

Let's destroy down the time period post-inflammatory hyperpigmentation. The prefix post- approach "after." Inflammatory is fairly self-explanatory, something that reasons irritation -- redness, swelling, and agony. Appears like a natural pimple, right?

Hyper- way "over" or "excessive." Pigmentation refers to the color of the dead .

So, altogether, postinflammatory hyperpigmentation literally method "immoderate color after inflammation."

whilst the skin repairs itself as a pimple heals, it might make too much melanin (the substance that gives your skin its color). The outcome is spot that's darker than the encircling skin . It's the dead 's average response to inflammation.

And it's no longer just pimples that purpose publish-inflammatory hyperpigmentation. Any injury, wound or infection can intent post-inflammatory hyperpigmentation to increase -- cuts and scrapes, burns, rashes and, yes, pimples.

Take heart in the knowledge that, whilst incredibly traumatic, these darkish spots are absolutely common. Virtually every man or woman with acne will improve submit-inflammatory hyperpigmentation to some measure.

PIH impacts both men and women equally, however it's extra common (and longer lasting) in darker skin tones. It impacts both men and females equally. Post-inflammatory hyperpigmentation isn't a true scar, and it is not invariably permanent.

Post-inflammatory hyperpigmentation is entirely a beauty difficulty. But post-inflammatory hyperpigmentation is disturbing;

some individuals in finding it more bothersome that genuine pimples. PIH on the whole fades, all on its possess, over time. There are also a lot of therapy choices to be had that may aid fade these pesky darkish spots turbo.

Your pimples is clearing up and your skin is looking higher day-to-day. However then you notice dark crimson or brown spots for your skin the place the acne lesions have healed. Is it scarring? And what are you able to do about it?

What is post-Inflammatory Hyperpigmentation?

Submit-inflammatory hyperpigmentation, or PIH, is the scientific time period given to discoloration of the skin that follows an inflammatory wound. It's the dead 's ordinary response to infection.

Put up-inflammatory hyperpigmentation looks like a flat subject of discoloration on the dead (these flat, discolored areas are also known as macules.) it will probably range in colour from crimson to crimson, pink, brown or black, relying for your skin tone and depth of the discoloration.

PIH develops when a scrape, rash, pimple, or other wound reasons your skin to come to be inflamed. Because the dead   heals, it frequently produces an excessive amount of melanin. Melanin is the protein within the skin that offers the skin its colour.

It is the surplus melanin that darkens and discolors the dead . This discoloration remains even after the wound or rash has healed.

Lamentably, PIH is very normal in those with pimples. It may well improve in all dead varieties, nevertheless it's extra long-established in darker dead tones. It influences each men and ladies equally.

PIH and acne

inflamed acne typically leave PIH spots behind after they heal. And it can be no longer simply the significant blemishes that cause these spots.

PIH macules can follow even rather minor acne and papules.

Nevertheless, the more infected a breakout, the higher and darker the PIH macule tends to be. Settling on or popping a pimple raises the chance of developing publish-inflammatory hyperpigmentation, effortlessly in view that you are growing irritation.

Treating PIH

submit inflammatory hyperpigmentation is not a scar within the genuine feel of the phrase. It might fade away over time, even without treatment. But it may take a very long time -- from a few weeks to 24 months to wholly fade.

The size of time it takes for PIH to fade depends on how darkish the PIH macule is in comparison with your skin tone. The bigger the contrast between the macule and your traditional dead tone, the longer it's going to take to fade.

Some post-inflammatory hyperpigmentation spots last longer, although, and will also be everlasting. There are cure options to be had to help fade even the most cussed put up-inflammatory hyperpigmentation spots.

First, although, your acne will have to be extra-or-much less underneath control earlier than starting any medication for PIH. In any other case, every new pimple would rationale a further PIH macule, decreasing the effectiveness of cure.

Anything healing option you select, have an understanding of that improvement will take time. Consider in terms of months as an alternative than weeks.

Additionally, many dermatologists endorse utilising a large-spectrum sunscreen day-to-day.

The solar may darken the discolorations and develop fading time.

Over-the-Counter remedies

mild instances of submit inflammatory hyperpigmentation can reply good to over-the-counter products. There is a plethora of "brightening" cure products on the market today.

Seem for a blend of alpha and beta hydroxy acids (including glycolic acid), diet A, nutrition C, and different constituents to exfoliate the dead . Other OTC ingredients that could be worthwhile are N-acetyl glucosamine and niacinamide.

Hydroquinone

Hydroquinone is a commonly used remedy for post inflammatory hyperpigmentation. It's on hand over-the-counter at 1% to 2% force, and in three% to 4% prescription lotions. Hydroquinone works via blocking the enzyme liable for melanin construction, thereby lightening the skin .

Hydroquinone lotions quite often incorporate additional lightening ingredients, reminiscent of kojic acid, glycolic acid, tretinoin and different retinoids, or nutrition C. These combo lotions can offer you better outcome than using hydroquinone on my own.

Hydroquinone lotions must be cautiously applied to darkened areas only, to restrict the unwanted lightening of your usual dead color. Hydroquinone may just rationale dead irritation for some persons. It is worth speaking to your health care professional before opening hydroquinone medication.

Topical Retinoids

Retinoids, similar to tretinoin and tazarotene, are probably prescribed to deal with acne. Retinoids help clear acne with the aid of dashing up cellphone turnover charges.

This speedy exfoliation may additionally aid clear PIH. Retinoid creams comprise Retin-A, Tazorac, and Differin. The truth that they scale back put up inflammatory hyperpigmentation as they deal with acne breakouts is an added bonus.

Obvious results may not be obvious for a couple of weeks to several months after commencing treatment. Also, be in search of excessive dryness, redness, and inflammation. This will trigger publish-inflammatory hyperpigmentation on its own.

Glycolic Acid

Glycolic acid is an alpha hydroxy acid found in lots of skin care merchandise. It simply exfoliates the skin , serving to to lighten submit inflammatory hyperpigmentation. To be had in cleansers, lotions, and gels, glycolic acid now not best helps enhance postinflammatory hyperpigmentation, but additionally leaves your skin tender and gentle.

Cleansers, gels, pads, and lotions containing glycolic acid are to be had over-the-counter. Higher concentrations are available with a prescription handiest. As with every merchandise, improvement may not be visible for a couple of months. Screen your skin   for irritation, and let your surgeon know if it occurs.

Azelaic Acid

Azelaic acid is used to treat pimples as well as PIH. To be had via prescription only, azelaic acid works by means of lowering infection and dashing up telephone turnover charges. Some experiences have shown azelaic acid to be as amazing as hydroquinone at treating hyperpigmentation. It is a good replacement for many who could also be unable to use hydroquinone.

Azelaic acid is to be had in cream and gel type and is frequently used along with glycolic acid or tretinoin.

As consistently, monitor your skin for redness and irritation and let your medical professional comprehend right away if you happen to expertise these side effects.

Procedural treatments

extra chronic instances of publish inflammatory hyperpigmentation may also be treated professionally at dead spas, medi-spas, or your dermatologist's place of work. Procedural cures comprise quite a lot of chemical peels and microdermabrasion. A sequence of remedies is required to safely fade PIH. Your health practitioner can help check which of these remedies, if any, could be correct for you.

Cortisone shots for acne is it just right for you ?

Every body hates those colossal, monster blemishes. They're big, painful, and take (what looks like) eternally to depart. Don't you wish you could magically make them disappear, or at the least heal extra speedily?

Although now not rather as wonderful as a magic wand, cortisone shots may be the following great factor. Accomplished for your dermatologist's place of job, this cure speedily reduces irritation, flattens and heals the breakout in only a few days.

The technical term for this system is intralesional corticosteroid injection, but many acne sufferers just name them steroid photographs, cortisone injections, or cyst injections.

How Cortisone pictures Work

Intralesional corticosteroid injections are used to deal with deep papules, nodules or cysts. An extraordinarily dilute corticosteroid is injected immediately into the blemish.

Don't fear, it can be a small needle! It is rapid and virtually painless.

The cortisone reduces infection particularly quickly. Over the following few days, you can discover your blemish softening and pulling down out. Most lesions heal within every week after cure.

And cure those big acne   speedily is not strictly for appears -- it also lessens the threat that the blemishes will rationale scars. This is in particular valuable if you are prone to scarring or hyperpigmentation.

Corticosteroid injections are also used to help reduce hypertrophic and keloid scars that you may have already got.

Viable side results

If too much cortisone, or too strong a dilution is used, the fat around the injection web site can atrophy. You'll become aware of depressions, or pitting, of the skin in the subject.

Fortunately, these depressions as a rule go away. This will take a very long time, although (up to 6 months). In many instances, this loss of tissue is everlasting.

By the way, should you boost everlasting pitting of the skin, it isn't necessarily brought on with the aid of the injections. Extreme breakouts customarily purpose atrophic scars. Dermal fillers is also a just right resolution in these cases.

Cortisone photographs Heal existing acne, but will not clear up Your acne

Cortisone injections have a lot of advantages, however there is one thing they just are not able to do -- resolve your acne . True, they support huge breakouts heal up quickly, but they can not discontinue extra breakouts from forming.

For that, you'll must use a daily acne remedy medication. Your dermatologist will prescribe a cure that's first-class to your skin. Some choices: topical retinoids, mixture acne medications, or even isotretinoin (relying on how severe your pimples is).

Except you most effective get a random large zit very sometimes, you can want a prescription acne remedy. For those significant blemishes, over-the-counter pimples products simply should not have enough oomph.

Utilizing an acne treatment every day stops breakouts from forming so, ideally, you is not going to want cortisone injections in any respect anymore.

Acne surgical procedure techniques and the way They help Your skin

The phrase surgical procedure brings up portraits of being wheeled into an surgical room the place an anesthesiologist is waiting for us, then waking up hours later with out a recollection of the entire method.

So, acne surgery could conjure up some frightening graphics. Is acne truly that severe that it requires surgical procedure?

Fairly, acne surgical procedure is a term that is used to describe a number of acne treatment approaches -- and none of them relatively as horrifying as your imagination might lead you to feel.

The methods are not your first line of security against pimples. Rather, they are used to deal with cussed breakouts that are not bettering with other therapies. Ordinarily, you'll be able to nonetheless use an acne remedy medicine furthermore to you acne surgical procedure process.

All of those therapies will also be achieved at your dermatologist's administrative center, and at some clinical spas.

Blemish Excision

Some blemishes are further stubborn and do not wish to respond to the medicines your health practitioner has prescribed. In this case, you dermatologist could determined that blemish excision will likely be worthy.

Excision is more commonly what most folks assume when they suppose "acne surgical procedure." A small incision is made within the skin , and the dermatologist drains the pus and particles from the blemish. You're conscious the entire time.

Ideally, after the pus is cleared, the blemish starts to heal. The system itself may just intent a mild scar, so you'll have got to come to a decision along with your health care provider if this is proper healing for you.

Extractions are just a little exceptional -- they're used to dispose of non-inflamed blemishes like blackheads and milia. An esthetician can deal with extractions for you.

Excision and extractions don't discontinue new breakouts from forming, although. They simply work on current blemishes. You'll nonetheless need to use an acne healing medication to get breakouts beneath manipulate.

These tactics are exceptional left to the scientific authorities. Do not ever attempt to lance and drain any blemish, tiny or now not. You open your self up to contamination and could easily scar your skin .

Laser surgical procedure

there are various special forms of laser treatments. They kind that's satisfactory for you depends on many explanations, like your skin style and colour, and what your ultimate goal is.

For the duration of a laser medication, a high depth pulse of light is directed onto the skin. Depending on the treatment used, laser can curb irritation and acne -causing bacteria, support existing pimples heal, and stimulates the skin to rejuvenate itself.

Lasers are used to treat each pimples and pimples scars. Some lasers want only one remedy to do the job, even as others require a few cures.

Laser cures are high priced, and ordinarily don't seem to be included via coverage.

Chemical surgical procedure

extra most likely referred to as chemical peels. You may be aware of the superficial or "lunchtime" peels which can be offered at your regional day spa. These peels gently exfoliate and haven't any downtime, despite the fact that your skin could also be a little bit red in a while.

Superficial peels are first-rate for treating slight acne .

Enhanced, medium-depth and deep chemicial peels are on hand at your dermatology workplace. There are one of a kind types of chemical peels, too. Your dermatologist will support you come to a decision which is pleasant on your skin .

All peel approaches are clearly the identical, though. A chemical agent is utilized to the skin and left for a period of time. The chemical removes the surface of the dead , triggering a transforming process. Over the subsequent a number of days to weeks, your skin will flake or "peel" off, allowing the renewed skin to return to the surface.

Identical to laser remedies, chemical peels can be used to treat each pimples and scarring.

Intralesional Injections

Intralesional corticosteroid injections, or what most of us effectively name cortisone injections, are additionally more often than not lumped into the acne surgery category. Cortisone injections are used to support scale back down significant, inflamed blemishes.

The dermatologist injects a small amount of cortisone instantly into the pimple. It sounds worse than it's, the needle used is particularly tiny. Over the direction of a few hours, the blemish flattens out.

Keep in mind cortisone injections an "emergency therapy" for large acne . You can nonetheless must use a common acne healing to get acne cleared up.

Will have to You See an Esthetician Or Dermatologist For acne

So you have determined to seek out a legit to support treat your acne. That's quality! Pimples will also be rough to deal with on your possess, so bringing in a pro is always a excellent inspiration.

But you'll be uncertain whom to name. Would your acne be with no trouble managed with the support of a expert esthetician, or would you be at an advantage making an appointment with your dermatologist?

What's an Esthetician?

Estheticians, often referred to as skin care therapists, are informed to perform cosmetic strategies such as facials, physique remedies, and waxing.

Most haven't any scientific training, they usually are not able to prescribe acne medicines.

However estheticians can aid maintain skin well being via performing deep cleaning facials and exfoliation remedies, as well as extracting pore blockages.

Estheticians can advocate skin care merchandise for your skin style and propose over-the-counter pimples cures. A excellent esthetician can even teach you tips on how to accurately take care of your skin at home.

When to see an Esthetician

In targeted cases, an esthetician can help you treat acne. If your acne is often moderate, with only a few blemishes and blackheads here and there, an esthetician could be an excellent choice.

Your esthetician can provide you with a series of pimples healing facials. She will even extract, or cleanse out, non-inflammatory breakouts and blackheads. Getting these therapies carried out in general will help keep your pores clear and minimize breakouts. That is why some dermatologists propose normal facials (depending to your skin).

Want support picking out skin care products that is not going to clog your pores or aggravate pimples? An esthetician can help you do this too.

Preserve in mind, an esthetician isn't a necessity in the case of treating pimples. Recall your esthetician your skin care help procedure.

Next Steps:

Treating pimples with help from an Esthetician

what's a Dermatologist?

Dermatologists are medical doctors who specialize within the remedy of the dead . Your dermatologist is a quality support in treating pimples. Not most effective will your dermatologist furnish quality dead care recommendation, she has a huge array of acne drugs -- both topical and systemic -- at her disposal.

There are matters an esthetician are not able to do for pimples. That is the place a dermatologist is precious.

When to look a Dermatologist

I've determined most humans struggle to know precisely when to name a dermatologist about their acne. On account that pimples is so usual, we tend to think it's no longer "severe ample" to carry in a health care provider.

But acne can extensively impact your skin, not to point out your great of existence. In case your acne is not responding to responding to over-the-counter treatments, or it's getting worse, regardless of cure, it's time to see a dermatologist.

Moderate to extreme inflammatory pimples consistently warrants a go back and forth to the dermatologist. Irrespective of how well you deal with your skin , you can doubtless want a prescription acne remedy to get this variety of pimples cleared up.

And if you would like recommendation or steerage in treating your pimples, it can be invariably a just right thought to call a dermatologist.

Now that you already know the best professional for you, what are you waiting for? Make that call right now. You'll be so blissful that you simply did!

Methods to handle buttocks pimples ?

Once we feel skin care we regularly suppose of our face. But the skin on our body needs some love, too! Primarily once we're dealing with body breakouts.

Acne can pop up all over the place: the again, chest, shoulders, even on the butt. But pimples can also be treated, regardless of the place it develops.

This article is all about find out how to take care of your acne - susceptible dead – developing the perfect cleaning and moisturizing routine (that is not going to irritate breakouts).

For support with physique acne remedies, pop over to these articles:

Treating again and physique pimples

get rid of Butt acne

Over-the-Counter physique acne cures

Now, learn on to create the ultimate physique care activities for acne -susceptible dead .

Grasp an acne-fighting physique cleaner.

Mild body breakouts ordinarily reply good to over-the-counter medicated physique washes, so that you could wish to there. Merchandise like Neutrogena body Clear physique Wash and

Phisoderm Anti-Blemish physique Wash incorporate salicylic acid, which is just right for bumps and blackheads.

Inflamed blemishes are inclined to reply higher to OTC benzoyl peroxide merchandise, like PanOxyl Foaming Wash or cleaning Bar. These merchandise can stain your washcloths and towels, although.

If you happen to're already using a health care provider prescribed acne medicine, you can also wish to forgo the medicated washes for a tender, all-over body purifier. Dove or Cetaphil are excellent non-drying and non-annoying manufacturers.

Ask your dermatologist if you should utilize a medicated or non-medicated physique wash.

Exfoliate, but gently.

Sure, it's main to maintain your skin exfoliated. However there's no ought to scrub the highest layer off of your body.

Body pimples are not able to be scrubbed away. Correctly, full of life scrubbing of the dead exacerbates infection of the follicles and can worsen breakouts.

A soft shower puff, washcloth or gentle body brush is all you need. Apply a squirt of physique wash and gently (gently) buff the skin. Tremendous abrasive scrubs and loofahs can do more damage than excellent, so steer clear.

In case your pimples is above all infected, pass the scrubbing altogether. You'll additional irritate breakouts.

Try baths instead of showers.

It is a excellent replacement to scrubbing. Soaking in a warm tub helps loosens useless skin cells. Keep in mind this a gentler strategy to slough away mobile particles and aid maintain the pores open and clear.

Some estheticians propose putting a cup of Epsom or lifeless Sea salt into the bathtub water to support heal infected lesions (it's excellent for sore muscle mass too!) make sure the pimples-effected areas remain submerged below the water for no less than twenty minutes.

Bathe instantly after sweating.

Sweat isn't your skin's friend, at the least no longer while you're acne inclined. Sweat can worsen current breakouts, so shower ASAP after figuring out or sweating.

Go forward and use gentle, oil-free lotions in the event you're feeling dry.

Pimples medicines can surely dry out your skin , regardless of where on the physique.

Despite the fact that the skin on the body is ordinarily extra oily than dead on the face, and no more prone to dry out, it may occur (isotretinoin, any individual?)

if you need body lotion, prefer a tender oil-free brand. It's much less likely to clog your pores and exacerbate breakouts.

Ditch scented lotions for now. Sure, they scent powerful. But if your skin is already dried out out of your acne medications, fragranced lotions can be disturbing.

Apply your acne therapy products.

So, now that you've bought your body care events down, it's time to center of attention on remedy. Good dead care by myself mostly isn't sufficient to solve body acne , particularly in case your acne is very infected or wellknown.

Apply your acne cures after your skin is cleansed and totally dry. Whether you're making use of prescription medicinal drugs or OTC products, ensure you comply with the usage instructional materials.

Don't have a body acne remedy yet? Talk with a dermatologist. Your derm will aid you create a body pimples treatment plan with a view to work pleasant for you.

10 things You have to learn about Treating Teen pimples in Boys

Most teen boys get acne. It is a traditional part of being a youngster... But it sort of sucks.

If you're inclined to place in somewhat little bit of time smearing some stuff to your face, and just a little little bit of persistence ready for it to work, that you can get your acne under manipulate.

1

Separate reality From Fiction

Would you be amazed to be trained that acne isn't induced through a soiled face? Acne just isn't induced with the aid of foods like chocolate or French fries, both.

Some folks are just susceptible to pimples, and these explanations are out of your manage. It can be no longer your fault that you're breaking out. Figuring out what fairly explanations acne (and what does not) will support you focus on treatments that work.

2

these merchandise You See On tv don't Clear acne overnight

the excellent news is there are plenty of acne medication products available on the market today that in reality can clear the skin. But even essentially the most amazing acne remedies aren't going to clear the skin overnight. They will not even clear pimples in three days, contrary to what the television commercial says.

If you're watching for a good OTC acne healing, the most potent will incorporate benzoyl peroxide. Seem for that ingredient. It's going to take at least a few weeks earlier than you start to particularly become aware of a change to your skin. If you're sufferer, you will see improvement (just now not as swiftly as some products declare).

• Can acne Be Cured?

• robust Over-the-Counter products

• the way to opt for The correct OTC acne therapy

three

Over-the-Counter merchandise could no longer Be enough

if you've tried a ton of OTC products and you are still breaking out, it is time to name in for some aid. Your healthcare professional has a lot of prescription choices with the intention to aid you get your pimples beneath control.

You do not always must see a dermatologist. Your loved ones general practitioner has generally helped plenty of teenagers deal with acne. You will see your typical doc first (they may refer you to a dermatologist if needed.)

Prescription drugs are without doubt improved and regularly work rapid than over-the-counter treatments. And they work when OTC treatments haven't.

• Are Prescription medications proper for Me?

- Is It Time to peer a health care provider?

- Treating Teen pimples

four

do not pass Your cures

once you get your cures house, you definitely need to use them. Sorry, guys, but teen boys are infamous for forgetting to use their treatments. And if you're no longer using them, they aren't going to clear your skin .

I know you are busy, and utilising treatments is a hassle, and generally you simply flat-out omit. Utilizing these cures is most important, though, so try to do anything it takes to use them day-to-day. That could imply leaving them subsequent to your toothbrush to jog your reminiscence, or asking your parents to help remind you. Anything it takes, simply are attempting not to pass your therapies.

- certainly not overlook Your therapies again!

- Readers respond: How Do You bear in mind Your acne cures?

5

Use Your therapies thoroughly

no longer only do you have to don't forget to make use of your therapies, but you also need to use them thoroughly. I do know, it seems like a affliction. When you get into the addiction of utilising your cures, although, it really is not that unhealthy and does not take too much time.

Make certain precisely the best way to use your acne medications. That implies studying all instructional materials (although it seems obvious) and following the directions your physician offers you (ask when you've got questions).

• Are You Over-making use of Your medicinal drugs?

• do not just Spot treat

6

maintain Your skin day-to-day

even though pimples isn't triggered via no longer washing your face, that excess oil and filth that builds up for the period of the day is not going to help concerns. Sweat may also irritate the skin and make pimples worse. So a excellent skin care movements is major.

It most effective takes a few minutes and also you don't want a ton of fancy products. Just a common face cleaning soap or cleanser and a moisturizer (if your skin is feeling dry) it's all you need.

• How in general must I Wash My Face?

• dead Care hints only for Guys

7

be careful To now not Shave pimples

Shaving is another subject. If you have acne in the beard subject, shave carefully. Go round them if in any respect feasible. Or at the least attempt to prevent shaving the tops off of your acne .

The extra you irritate your skin , the more purple and inflamed it is going to look. The dead on the face can be touchy, so try to treat it gently. This will imply shaving less customarily, as a minimum unless your pimples isn't so inflamed

8

body acne can also be handled Too

The face isn't the only situation that pimples can pop up. You would get acne to your chest, again, shoulders and neck. It happens; it is long-established.

The various identical drugs which might be used for the face are also used for the physique. Benzoyl peroxide soaps and physique washes are probably used to deal with physique breakouts. Your health practitioner would additionally prescribe different medications, like oral antibiotics or even isotretinoin (Accutane), relying on how critical the breakouts are.

9

persist with It

no matter what healing you are making use of -- whether it's whatever you received from your physician or the drugstore -- you have to keep on with it long ample for it to work.

It takes a very long time for a treatment to work. Stick with your treatment for no less than 8-10 weeks before identifying if it is working or now not. Do not jump from therapy to cure. And assume to get new acne for the period of this time, too. They won't discontinue suddenly, however as a substitute slowly start fading away.

Don't stop once your skin   clears, either. Pimples medicinal drugs don't discontinue acne   for excellent; they only hold it below manage. So if you happen to discontinue making use of the remedy, acne will most of the time come correct again (the exception here would be isotretinoin/Accutane). At some point, your acne will go away on its possess and you can sooner or later be competent to get rid of your acne therapies for excellent. Unless then, stick with it.

• Why aren't My treatments Working?

• Why Did My pimples Come again?

• Teen acne cure pointers

10

pimples can make You think unhealthy, however which you can Beat It

you may not need to admit it to anybody, but pimples can take a toll to your self-esteem. It will probably make you think much less positive, insecure, indignant, and depressed. These are average feelings.

Establishing with healing and seeing some good results can support you instantly believe higher. So can focusing on matters rather than your skin (physical activities, tune, art, or any other interests you have).

But sometimes you just can not seem to no longer think about your pimples. If pimples is controlling more of your existence than you need it to, let any one comprehend. Tell your dad and mom, a favourite trainer or clergy man or woman, your doctor, someone you trust.

Pimples is a ordinary a part of being a teenager. Which you could get through it, that you can recover from it, and you could believe good about your skin and your self once more.

10 matters Teen girls should learn about acne

lots of sweet sixteen women have acne . But realizing you have got manufacturer nonetheless would not make you think significantly better about your own skin, does it?

You do not ought to wait until you "develop out of" pimples. With a while and the proper cure, you'll be able to be amazed at how much which you can beef up your skin .

1

You did not do anything to motive your pimples

pimples is not your fault. It is brought on by many matters, all of that are out of your manipulate.

So it's not the chocolate bar you ate last night, or the pizza and soda you had over the weekend. It can be no longer in view that you're now not cleansing your face properly. And it's not your make-up (mostly).

When it comes right down to it, it's the hormonal changes that occur during puberty. And some individuals are just going to get pimples; it can be on your genes. So do not feel guilty—you failed to do whatever to intent your pimples.

2

these products you see on tv don't particularly work in a single day

you realize what i am speakme about, proper? Some young adults, or even celebrities, speaking about how such and such product started clearing their skin "from the second I put it on" or how their "breakouts cleared up in a single day." it can be so tempting!

These acne products may just really be robust and would remedy your skin , however none work overnight. Nothing can clear acne that quick, it doesn't matter what the commercials say.

For an amazing OTC medication, appear for person who has benzoyl peroxide. These may also be the products from tv, or you will discover benzoyl peroxide products at the store too (they mainly price much less and work just as well.)

Then, use these products for eight-10 weeks before expecting to see a difference on your skin.

3

You might ought to see a doctor about your pimples

If these OTC merchandise are not doing a lot for you, a prescription treatment perhaps the trick. This means a shuttle to your health practitioner.

I know you would on the whole as an alternative deal with acne in your own with products you to find on the store or salon, but generally OTC merchandise are not rather robust ample. On this case, you can be so much happier with a prescription medicine, above all whenever you start seeing results.

Pimples is so customary in teenagers, your loved ones surgeon or pediatrician more than likely has expertise treating it. Your doc can prescribe an pimples medication medicine, or refer you on to a dermatologist.

Do not wait; the sooner you begin medication, the earlier you'll be able to see development.

4

You need to use your remedies everyday

So you've got your remedies all set, whether or not they are OTC or prescription. Now you ought to use them!

Looks like a no brainer, however absolutely it is easier than you consider to forget your medicines. You rush out of the condominium in the morning for institution, or you spend the night at a buddy's residence and depart your cures at dwelling. You've got tons of activities and interests that maintain you on the go. Acne therapies can quite simply be forgotten about.

The more regular you might be with making use of your treatments, the better results you are going to see. So do your excellent to not pass a dose.

Set your telephone cellphone to alarm at remedy time, ask your mum and dad to remind you, depart a sticky word on the replicate, something to get you utilizing your medications daily.

5

You need to use your therapies adequately

do you know the most usual reason why acne   therapies do not work? It's not due to the fact they don't seem to be strong; it is that they aren't getting used thoroughly.

Be certain you're utilising your treatments effectively: do not spot deal with, don't over-apply, and don't bounce round between treatments. Stick with something lengthy enough to see results, and use it consistently.

Read all of the directions to your medicinal drugs, and ask your surgeon if you have any questions.

6

Be patient; acne takes time to deal with

Even when you are doing the whole lot right, it takes time to look results—about eight-12 weeks. That is a very long time when you're relatively desperate for clear skin .

It may look like, as a minimum to start with, your products are not working at all. You are ancient acne is not going to fade tremendous speedy, and you'll be able to still get some new acne .

It's frustrating and you'll think like giving up. Do not! Preserve using your therapies even supposing you do not see outcome right away.

7

make-up is okay, just wash it off at night

while you are waiting on your acne to remedy, that you can cover it up if you want to. Sure, that you can wear makeup even though you may have pimples. It won't make pimples worse, provided that you select the correct makeup and ensure to scrub it off at night time.

Eight

ladies get physique pimples too (it is fully natural)

physique acne can make you suppose uncomfortable sporting tank tops, spaghetti straps, and swimsuits. Even finding a prom costume can also be an exercise in frustration you probably have body pimples.

Here is a little bit secret—lots of girls have physique breakouts, and it can be dealt with.

 With a body wash or bar containing benzoyl peroxide (5 percent-10 percentage strength). Use that everyday for a couple of weeks.

When you don't seem to be seeing results, talk to your healthcare professional. Physique acne can be stubborn, so a prescription medication is more commonly a just right concept.

9

you'll be able to have got to use pimples cures even after your skin clears up

Yay! Your skin has cleared up! However don't stop using your remedies yet.

You'll customarily have got to hold utilising your treatments even after your skin has cleared up. This doesn't mean the treatment failed to work properly. Pimples remedies do not healing acne, they only manipulate it. In the event you stop utilising them, acne will come back.

Isotretinoin, also known as Accutane, is one exception. This medicine is not used lengthy-time period, and acne probably would not come back.

So, plan on sticking together with your cure for a even as. Ultimately, your skin will discontinue breaking out on its possess and you'll be ready to discontinue therapies for excellent. Unless then, simply work with it.

10

Feeling down? There is hope and help

acne could make you believe depressed, indignant, hopeless. It will probably affect your self-self assurance and your vainness. It may be difficult to confess that acne has that a lot manage over us, but your feelings are normal.

Try to focal point on things that make you consider good about your self. Might be you are a nice artist or softball participant, talented musician, or budding fashionista. Don't forget these matters you adore about yourself.

Speakme to someone else can also support. Definite, you can also consider a bit of embarrassed in the beginning to be speakme about your skin problems, however people who are practically you and love you are going to appreciate.

Talk to your parents, your first-rate buddy, a favourite teacher, relative, or clergy man or woman. This is chiefly proper should you think like acne is overwhelming your existence.

Although having teen pimples is difficult, you could get through this period for your existence. Just opening on an acne cure could make you think more in manipulate and positive

simple tips for Treating Teen pimples

practically every body battles teen acne at some factor. Get some teen acne remedy recommendations to help you together with your skin -clearing hobbies.

Take good care of your skin daily.

Despite the fact that acne isn't precipitated with the aid of no longer washing your face, excellent skin care is still an essential step on your pimples healing events. Use a foaming cleaner each morning and night, preferably one with benzoyl peroxide or salicylic acid. A light, oil-free moisturizer can be utilized if acne therapies make your skin believe tight, or you've got flaking or peeling.

For physique acne , use a medicated physique wash. Shower as quickly as viable after sweating or working out, when you consider that sweat can irritate acne breakouts. Do not scrub the skin too difficult both. Whether or not acne is in your face or body, scrubbing can broaden inflammation and is not going to help clear breakouts rapid. You're treating your skin very gently, enabling it to heal.

Be regular with your remedies.

Ultra-modern young adults are tremendous busy, so it may be tough to recollect to use your acne therapies. But if you want excellent outcome you ought to be steady, because of this making use of your treatment medicines daily as directed. Try to not skip days.

In case you have quandary remembering your medications, placing them in a place that you'll be able to effortlessly see them is a straightforward reminder. Using your medicines whilst every day may also keep you from forgetting about them. You too can want to leave yourself a word, or ask your moms and dads to remind you.

Too much of a excellent thing is… an excessive amount of.

Consistency is excellent, however do not over-do your pimples therapies. Applying topical therapies too mostly or utilizing too much at a time is not going to clear your pimples any faster. What you're going to get is purple, peeling dead . Do not provide in to this temptation. As hard as it is, be sufferer and provides the medicinal drugs some time to work.

Along the equal lines, do not over-cleanse your face both. Despite the fact that thorough cleansing can maintain dead   from feeling too oily, immoderate cleaning may also be aggravating to the skin . Hold your cleansing down to simply two or 3 times daily. Your skin will feel easy with out feeling stripped or over-dried.

Keep your fingers off your face.

Don't squeeze, select, pop, or poke at your pimples. You are able to do tremendous harm to your skin , and motive scarring. While you squeeze a pimple, you place numerous stress on the follicle wall. If this wall breaks, contaminated material can spread underneath the skin. Skin tissue may also be irreparably damaged.

Even though pus drains from the pimple, injury can nonetheless be occuring beneath the skin 's surface where you can not see.

Do not forget, that pimple is just transitority, but a scar can final forever. It can be not worth popping that zit. Apart from, more commonly squeezing a pimple leaves it larger and redder than it used to be before. If it is fairly bothering you, use a spot therapy on it alternatively.

Use the proper makeup.

When you have acne , it's natural to need to cover them up. But making use of comedogenic make-up will most effective make your pimples worse. Heavy makeup and oil-founded foundations can purpose a type of acne referred to as pimples cosmetica.

For those who do put on make-up, decide upon an oil-free manufacturer that's labeled noncomedogenic or nonacnegenic. And always thoroughly cleanse every hint of make-up away with a foaming purifier every night time. By no means go to sleep with makeup on. You too can wish to go away your skin naked as a lot as viable.

Start on a tested pimples remedy.

Yes, odds are you'll outgrow your pimples. But that does not mean you must, or will have to, wait except that day comes.

There are plenty of relatively just right therapies out there that may help remedy the breakouts you have got now, and discontinue new acne from forming. Which you could with acne products that you simply purchase at the store, and progress to prescription cures if these do not work.

Anything you do, though, do not put matters on the dead that are not imply for the dead . There are numerous bizarre "healing" strategies on the internet (or instructed by means of your neighbors) that you should steer clear of.

Matters like toothpaste, Windex, milk of magnesia, or urine will not work for acne , and they very well could cause a ton of issues for your skin .

Speak to your moms and dads about getting medication to your pimples.

In case your pimples is not improving with over-the-counter therapies, ask for aid. Your pediatrician or household general practitioner can deal with teenage acne , so you may also now not even desire a referral to peer a dermatologist.

Consider, your acne will also be cleared, if you are willing to be patient and treat it right.

Top smart ways to treat acne for tuition students

You've left excessive institution in the back of, so why is acne still putting around?

It more commonly received't make you consider a lot better, nevertheless it's original for university-aged students to have acne . Lots of humans to find their teenage acne hangs on into their institution years.

And even supposing you've managed to get by means of excessive college with rather clear skin , pimples could shock you by doping up for the first time now.

Pimples is disturbing, but that you may get it below control. It simply takes a bit of of time, endurance, and some know-how.

Newly breaking out? Are trying an OTC pimples medicine.

Pimples customarily appears during the school years. School is fundamental time for acne breakouts. It is now not uncommon for pimples to show up for the first time throughout your late teens and early twenties.

If your skin has been rather resolve until this factor, and you are just coping with slight acne or occasional breakouts and blemishes, over-the-counter acne cures may be just what you need.

Now not just any product off the shelf will do, though. The most potent ones include benzoyl peroxide. Assess the ingredient label.

And do not worry about shopping the most high-priced product. Familiar manufacturers work simply as good, and fit inside your university scholar finances.

Already on an pimples remedy? Take them with you.

Everybody perpetually told you that you'd outgrow your pimples whenever you graduated high university. Sadly, acne would not care what age you're. It is probably acne with comply with you to institution.

That is why it is predominant to take your acne medicinal drugs with you as you head off to university, and be certain you may have a plan to continue getting your prescriptions whilst you are faraway from dwelling.

Lots of young adults make a decision to stop utilizing their pimples cures at this age. Even supposing your skin appears good and clear now, it can be the treatments which might be keeping it that approach. Stop making use of your medications, and pimples is more likely to come back.

Continuously use your acne therapies.

Classes, learning, work, and looking to have a existence... It can be rough to fit it all in. It is super easy to overlook to make use of your pimples cures every day. Plus, parents mainly don't seem to be round to remind you anymore!

Pimples cures best work if they are used very always. Skipping doses or forgetting days will come again to hang-out you.

Definite, it is tempting to wish to simply fall into bed after an extended day. And it is convenient to bypass treatments when you're rushing to get to type on time in the morning (or pulling an all-night be trained session.)

Most people feel their treatments are not working, when in all reality they are not utilising them as they will have to. So, in case you rather need to see growth on your skin you might have Got to make utilizing your treatments a priority.

Aid! I preserve Forgetting to use My acne remedies

do not hold your hopes on residence therapies.

Acne healing recommendation appears to run rampant on college campuses. From kitchen remedies, like garlic and apple cider vinegar, to the extra weird milk of magnesia or urine, it seems like every person has their own "definite-fireplace" alleviation to share.

As tempting as it could be to give these a are trying (good enough, urine isn't all that tempting) there aren't any house cures which were established mighty towards pimples.

At exceptional, you can waste time trying treatments which might be never going to work. At worst, you'll be able to grow to be with a nasty case of contact dermatitis from striking stuff for your face that was in no way meant to your face.

Seriously, do yourself a desire and skip these cures. Use merchandise which might be principally made to treat acne .

Pimples is not all that handy to treat, as you're most of the time discovering out. If you've tried to care for it on your possess without so much good fortune, or in case your pimples is really inflamed, painful, or extreme, have a surgeon take a seem.

For those who're still to your dad and mom' wellness coverage, making an appointment is most likely less difficult. But if no longer, see if your student health core can direct you to a hospital. Even though you can not see a dermatologist correct away, a basic observe health practitioner can nonetheless support get you started on medication.

Do not wait! Pimples doesn't have to control your institution years. That you could get it cleared.

Dead Sea Mud Face Masks at Home: How to Use Dead Sea Mud Masks

Enjoy spa-quality Dead Sea Mud face masks at home! Every day when you simply wash your face, you disturb the natural mantel of the skin, causing redness and an uneven tone. Regular use of a Dead Sea Mud face mask at home

Each day when you simply wash your face

• You disturb the natural mantel of the skin, causing redness and uneven tone

• Dead Sea Mud helps restore pH levels, removing the red face look

• Minerals in Dead Sea Mud feed the skin nutrients, keeping it hydrated and giving it less wrinkle retention

• A Dead Sea Mud mask leaves your skin with a glow of youthfulness and cleanliness.

• Dead Sea Mud moisturizes your skin and helps with natural skin hydration

Why use a dead sea mud mask?

Why use a dead sea mud mask, you ask? The answer is because authentic, 100% pure Dead Sea Mud is, hands-down, one of the best skin care ingredients in nature, particularly so for anyone with adult acne and/or mature skin who are looking to turn back the hands of time and purify the skin of all the toxins and dirt that can get lodged in the pores. It contains 26 natural minerals, which act like vitamins for your skin, and many of which can be found only in the waters of the Dead Sea. Dead Sea Mud is also a great alternative to a chemical peel.

Who is this mask best for?

Authentic, 100% pure Dead Sea Mud is an extremely rich and powerful deep cleanser and anti-aging spa treatment, so ideally it is for any of the following groups:

• Men and women over 30

• Oily and/or acnetic skin

• Mature skin

Those younger than 30 with acne or who wish to deep cleanse their facial pores may wish to try our Dead Sea Mud Soap instead, which contains the highest concentrations of pure, authentic Dead Sea Mud you'll likely ever see in a mud bar, but not so much that it will overwhelm your youthful skin. Those with dry/dehydrated skin or sensitive skin may also wish to try our mud bar in lieu of our mud mask. Use our mud bar daily or weekly to wash your face. All your pores will be perfectly cleaned.

What can The Castle Baths mud mask do for you?

Castle Baths' Dead Sea Mud Mask will deep-cleanse your pores, where ordinary cleansers cannot reach, and draw out all the toxins, dirt, and dead skin cells that have been building up over time and dulling your natural radiance. It will infuse your skin with 26 unique natural minerals, which act like vitamins and feed your skin with all the nutrients it needs to preserve youthful elasticity, and it will moisturize your entire face, all at the same time! Our Dead

Sea Mud Mask gives you spa quality results in less than half an hour from the comfort of your home!

Where can I get this mud mask?

This mud mask is sold exclusively through Castle Baths here on our website. You can purchase it here individually in 8 oz or 15 oz sizes or get it along with some of our other popular Tre'Yours skin care products by treating yourself to our Dead Sea Gift Basket.

Once my mud arrives, what should I do next?

Stir it up. if you feel its thick and you want it to last longer, try adding some dead sea brine to the mud. Our mud is 100% dead sea mud which by the way is the mud from the bottom of the dead sea with some of the actual dead sea water known as brine . So you can have really thick mud or even a thinner version based on your own preference.

How often should I use Dead Sea Mud?

• Use our mud mask weekly.

• Use our mud soap daily.

Important Information about using a Dead Sea Mud Mask

Directions and notations:

Always do a small skin test first to make certain your skin type can handle the strength of the mineral content and salt in this mud product. Many dead sea mud mask are diluted with water and or fillers, Castle Baths mud is pure and powerfully full of mineral content.

Use and Skin Type:

Use Tre'Yours Dead Sea Mud as a mask once or twice per week as needed. Apply a sparely thin layer on skin- Allow to slightly dry for 7-12 minutes and rinse well! If it takes longer than 15 minutes to slightly dry- you are using the mud too thick. If your skin type is dry or sensitive- do not use more than once per week. ALL Mask, especially mud, works best if it is rinsed before its 100% dry- in other words, rinse before the cracking stage!

- The Castle Baths mud has an interior seal on the jar , however we do not heat seal the seal...our seals are simply placed on the jar lid to protect the lid itself from the mud. Sometimes they self seal and sometimes they do not completely self seal.

FIRST

When you first open up your dead sea mud, if it has been sitting, the salty seas water will separate from the mud somewhat and float to the top. You should stir it back to a constancy mud base

Use on hair, face, and or body

1. Apply sparingly. Dead Sea Mud applied too thick will cause the mud to not dry properly.

2. If you have sensitive skin, or wax your upper lip area- do NOT mud this area!

3. Always apply on the face using upward strokes. Never pull the face skin downward. Gravity does enough of that for you.

4. Be gentle around the eye area. Be careful not to get the dead sea mud in your eyes

5. If the mud begins to feel dry or itchy- you need to rinse it off…it is finished doing what it is designed to do.

6. If you notice blemishes arise after using this mud you may need to wait a week and detox again due to the toxins in your pores being lifted and extracted.

7. The mud is not designed to remove blackheads in one use- you will need several applications. Please never pick blemishes or blackheads.

How to use Dead Sea Mud on the face or body:

-Apply a thin layer of mud to cleansed skin while gently massaging onto the skin with your fingers (be sure to keep the mud away from eyes and mouth).

-As you apply the mud, never use your fingers in a downward motion, apply with upward strokes. Gravity already does enough pulling of the face downward.

-Leave the mud on the skin for 7-12 minutes allowing the mud to slightly dry. If the mud begins to crack and itch- it has been on too long.

To remove mask:

For face- Use a wet lukewarm or cool soft wash cloth and lay on your face for a few seconds to soften the mask, then rinse the remaining mud off with warm water. Try not to scrub as you remove your mask,

For body- try hopping into a warm shower to rinse the mask.

How often should I apply a Dead Sea Mud mask to my skin?

Because of the incredibly high mineral and salt content of the Dead Sea Mud, it may affect individuals with different skin, differently depending on their skin type and sensitivities. Limit one application per week if you have dry or sensitive skin. Normal to oily skin types can apply 2 times a week if desired.

*Important -Because of the high mineral and salt content the mud may slightly tingle or sting the skin. If at any point the mud becomes uncomfortable, rinse off with warm water to remove the mask. If you feel burning or itching- rinse, don't wait.

Dead Sea/Black Mud Benefits for hair:

-Yes, the mud can cleanses hair and scalp while helping to remove dandruff mud leaves hair soft, with a healthy shine

How to use Dead Sea Mud/Black Mud as a hair mask:

-Massage mud to your scalp, and then work throughout your hair.

-Allow mask to set for up to 20 minutes before rinsing out thoroughly

Steps to show you how to use our Dead Sea Mud as a mask. Dead Sea Mud can be used on face, body, or hair

FIRST

When you first open up your dead sea mud, if it has been sitting, the salty seas water will separate from the mud somewhat and float to the top. You should stir it back to a constancy mud base.

NEXT

Stir your Dead Sea Mud thoroughly. Try using a butter knife for a nice, smooth consistency.

Your mud is now mixed and ready to go!

Dead Sea Mud is known for anti-aging, anti-wrinkles, deep cleansing, and is effective at helping to take away blackheads, white heads, fine lines, and helping to lighten freckles.

Use on hair, face, and or body

Ok, Now the Fun Part:

1. Apply sparingly. Dead Sea Mud applied too thick will cause the mud to not dry properly.

2. Use your finger tips, and small circular motions.

3. If you have sensitive skin, or wax your upper lip area- do NOT mud this area!

4. Always apply on the face using upward strokes. Never pull the face skin downward. Gravity does enough of that for you.

5. Be gentle around the eye area. Be careful not to get the dead sea mud in your eyes.

5. Wait 8-12 minutes or until mud is almost fully dry. You'll know the mud is dry by the tightness you will feel over the entire face.

6. Once the dead sea mud is almost fully dried, rinse completely off, either in the shower or from the sink.

Finish up with your make up for a beautiful mini facelift appearance. You will notice several of your deep lines lifted not as deep, and many of the fine lines lightened. The dead sea mud gently peels away dead skin cells to reveal a more youthful, healthier skin layer and outer glow.

Dead Sea Skin Care - use CB's Tre'Yours Mud Bar daily and CB's Tre'Yours Dead Sea Mud Mask weekly for best results - wash with our Dead Sea Mud Soap bar!

CB Tre'Yours Dead Sea Mud - with high concentration of minerals such as magnesium, calcium, bromide and potassium, the mud pampers the skin.

Dead Sea Mud Mask- How To Prepare It And What Are Its Benefits?

Did you know that a Dead Sea Mud Mask can help you get rid of acne and soothe skin ailments? Well, it's true! The mud found around Dead Sea, one of the biggest salt lakes in the world, is especially therapeutic, and it has many uses in soap and other cosmetic products around the world.

So, would you like to know how to use this mask to get glowing and flawless skin? Continue with your read!

Benefits Of Dead Sea Mud Mask:

Dead Sea mud has many amazing health benefits, which help refresh and revitalize your skin. Dead Sea mud reduces wrinkles, has emollient and anti-acne properties, and it is also used to ameliorate conventional medical therapy.

Apart from these amazing healths benefits, Dead Sea mud has some essential properties that help reduce and treat conditions like psoriasis, eczema, and acne. Soaps made with Dead Sea mud help cure itching, while they also cleanse the skin and remove dead skin.

Usually, you can add any essential oil to the Dead Sea mud face mask, but this recipe will use lavender, chamomile, and peppermint essential oils. Let's look at why these ingredients are the best possible additions to this face mask.

Ingredients Used In Dead Sea Mud Masks:

Lavender Essential Oil:

Lavender essential oil has a calm and soothing effect. It has been used in many cultures as a sleep aid. The especially alluring scent of lavender essential oil enchants most people. It is used widely by chemists and beauticians as an ingredient in lotions, gels and other body and face packs. Lavender oil not only helps reduce and relieve tension, but it also disinfects your skin. Lavender essential oil has been known to treat respiratory problems.

Chamomile Essential Oil:

This is another effective skin soothing essential oil. Its calm and naturally soothing effect helps you relax, while it also exhibits anti-inflammatory properties. Chamomile essential oil helps relax skin irritation like eczema and acne. You can even use it to reduce the irritation.

Peppermint Essential Oil:

This essential oil is mostly used in chewing gum, ice cream, tea, soap, and shampoo. Peppermint oil has many varied health benefits, which include the treatment of nausea, reducing headaches and clearing respiratory tract and respiratory problems. This essential oil is crammed with minerals and nutrients like iron, manganese, magnesium, folate, calcium, copper and potassium.

×

Dead Sea Mud Mask:

Now that you know about the benefits of Dead Sea Mud and other ingredients of this face mask, let's take a look at how you can make this incredible moisturizing mud mask for your face and your body:

The Ingredients:

To begin with you must gather your ingredients, obviously. These ingredients include:

• A glass jar with a lid

• ½ cup Dead Sea mud

• 1 drop peppermint essential oil

• 3 drops chamomile essential oil

• 4 drops lavender essential oil

• A mixing bowl

• Spoon

• Cloth

• Water

Directions:

Here is the Dead Sea mud mask recipe:

1. Pour the ½ cup Dead Sea mud in a mixing bowl.

2. Add the lavender, chamomile and peppermint essential oils to the mixing bowl.

3. Mix the ingredients well until you get a smooth paste.

4. Now pour the paste into the glass jar with the lid.

5. This face mask paste can now be stored and kept aside for further use.

6. Now that the mask paste is ready, take one tablespoon of this paste in your hands.

7. Using your first two fingers proceed to apply the paste evenly over your face.

8. Remember to avoid the delicate area around your eyes and mouth.

If your skin begins to get inflamed or get irritated remove the mask with water.

9. Once you have applied the mask, leave it on for 10 minutes.

10. Proceed to wipe it off using a gentle face cloth dipped in warm water.

Well, use these steps and make your own amazing Dead Sea mud face mask at home. Please tell us about any other recipe variations or your experiences using Dead Sea mud here. Leave a comment below.

Pimples Got You Down? : 5 methods to keep despair away and feel extra positive

acne bought you down? You're not by myself. It's traditional to think discouraged, even self-aware, when looking to clear a case of acne.

Taking good care of yourself gives you a rationale to believe just right about your body, and may offer you a carry whilst you want it most.

1

consume well.

Consuming a healthy food regimen is excellent to your body, and will finally help you consider better. Eating correct will supply your complete physique, including your skin , the vitamins and minerals it needs to remain healthy.

Are there any meals you will have to hinder in case you have acne ? Perhaps. A couple of small studies have proven a correlation between designated meals and acne severity. Dairy merchandise and excessive carb foods foods seem to be the worst offenders.

These foods do not always motive pimples in a in any other case clear-skinned person, but may irritate existing acne breakouts. So, if a meals seems to make your acne worse, avert that specified dish.

2

Get enough sleep.

Face it, the whole lot appears worse when you're tired and cranky. Try to get eight hours of sleep every night, or take common naps when you need them. When you're good rested it can be easier to hold things in viewpoint.

Just make sure you are cleaning your face before hitting the pillow every night time. Disposing of dirt, excess oil, and make-up will aid get your skin   into form, and aid you remember to apply those pimples therapies too.

three

exercise by and large.

One be trained suggests those with pimples are inclined to recreation lower than their clear-skinned counterparts. But recreation is a great way to strengthen your mood!

Now not simplest does ordinary exercise make your heart and lungs robust, but it helps you beat stress and might ease nervousness and depression. Apart from, whilst you feel just right concerning the things your physique can do, it lets you focal point much less to your skin.

Invariably bathe as quickly as viable after exercising, though. Sweat can also be stressful and worsen pimples, particularly

back and physique breakouts.

4

begin treating your acne, if you have not already.

Pimples is not going to go away on its possess, so the sooner you begin treatment the better.

If your acne is slight, are trying an over-the-counter product. However don't wait to peer a doctor if you are not seeing any development after a couple of weeks. Your healthcare professional has an arsenal of acne-combating treatments as a way to get you to your strategy to clearer skin.

It is convenient to think helpless when you are breaking out and don't know methods to discontinue it. Simply realizing you have got taken a step to reinforce your skin can aid you consider more in manipulate.

5

Get support, if you would like it.

Acne will also be an upsetting quandary, causing you to feel self-conscious or embarrassed. You're now not being useless. Many persons with acne feel the identical means you do.

Everyone has down days as soon as in a while. But when acne is impacting your lifestyles to the point that it's negatively affecting your self-esteem, it is time to get support. Speak to your medical professional. Do not disregard your feelings, and do not be ashamed.

Melancholy, anxiety, social withdrawal, and ideas of suicide are all warning indicators you shouldn't ignore. Please get support correct away. With support, which you could suppose better.

Beauty secrets OF CLEOPATRA

we'll speak about some beauty pointers that Queen Cleopatra took potential of:

1) Cleopatra's acne bathtub of almond oil and honey.

One of the crucial famous beauty secrets of Cleopatra used to be " almond oil and honey" pimples bath. Cleopatra used to combine recent honey and almond oil.

We will come what may imitate this beauty secret of "everlasting formative years" from the noted Queen. To organize the honey acne bath, mix half cup of honey with 5 tablespoons almond oil (you would use olive oil as an alternative), then pour this substance into your pimples bath take pride of soft and delicate skin !

2) physique scrub of beauty Queen:

For higher influence of the honey pimples bath, the servants of Cleopatra used to therapeutic massage her physique with amazing, common body scrub.

You are going to want: 2 desk spoons of sea salt and 3 table spoons of thick cream (average, flavour free cream).

Mix sea salt with cream and gently rub your physique with it in round motions. Ensure to go away this scrub to take a seat for your skin for at least 5 minutes, then rinse. This scrub will gently exfoliate your skin and make your physique suppose smooth and smooth like heaven!

3) Face cream of Cleopatra:

an extra beauty secret of Cleopatra is a targeted face cream.

You are going to need:

2 tablespoons of aloe vera juice,

4 drops of rose essential oil,

1 tablespoon of almond oil,

2 spoons of beeswax.

Slowly warmth the beeswax and almond oil till the substance will get liquid, but don't boil it (that you may differ the quantity of beeswax, the more of it you add – the thicker your cream will likely be). Add aloe vera juice and rose most important oil, mix wholly. (non-compulsory: that you can add diet E tablet into your cream).

Let your cream relax, pour it into a tumbler container and retailer on your fridge (it might probably last for roughly a week). All of the materials are utterly usual and filled with nutrients. Isn't it powerful!

Four) clean facial masks of Cleopatra:

one of the crucial noted beauty secrets of beautiful Queen Cleopatra used to be making facial masks utilizing white clay. Here is much like hers recipe you could prepare at residence utilising white clay, honey and olive oil (or almond oil).

Combine 2 desk spoons of white clay with 1 desk spoon of honey and 1 table spoon of olive oil. Observe this masks for your face for 10-15 minutes and then, rinse with warm water. (that you may store this masks in the fridge for a couple of days.) Your skin will consider amazingly refreshed and delicate.

5) Antiseptic nourishing masks of Cleopatra:

you'll want:

– 1 egg yolk

– 1 desk spoon of almond oil

– 1 tea spoon of honey

commercial

combine all of the ingredients collectively and apply it to your face for 10-15 minutes. This mask may be very refreshing and nourishing! Your skin will love it. (best be certain you aren't allergic to the parts of this mask)

6-Cleopatra's common beauty soap:

some of the magnificence secrets of Cleopatra is: she adored utilising oatmeal to cleanse her dead . Many soaps at the present time can be harsh and worsening for the dead , chiefly, for a touchy. Oatmeal can't only cleanse the skin, removing the dirt and rather exfoliating, but in addition, it's moisturizing and nourishing. To cleanse the dead   using an oatmeal – combine oats with warm water in a bowl and wait unless oats get soft, then, gently massage smooth oatmeal all over your face for approximately a minute (be certain that the temperature of your do-it-yourself soap is cozy to touch, we don't wish to be harsh making use of scorching oatmeal mass on our face); even as massaging, hinder eye area. Rinse your skin with heat after which, bloodless water and enjoy soft, cleansed and moisturized skin

.

7-Cleopatra's masks for cleansing and whitening the skin:

mix in a bowl 1 table spoon of white clay, 1 table spoon of honey and 1 desk spoon of lemon juice. Apply this mask to your face for roughly 10 minutes after which, rinse with warm water. Be detailed you are not allergic to any of the constituents earlier than making this do-it-yourself magnificence remedy.

This masks has antiseptic houses due to honey, lemon juice will help slightly whiten and brighten your skin   and also, this homemade facial mask will naturally hydrate and tighten your skin

.

Eight-

Renewing emulsion of Cleopatra:

Cleopatra invented this emulsion herself. This home made magnificence treatment can support renew and hydrate the skin , adding youthful glow to the face. To arrange this therapy you're going to desire a sterling silver bowl, pure thermal water, aloe Vera juice and honey.

Pour 1 cup of thermal water into a silver bowl, add 2 desk spoons of fresh aloe Vera juice (preferably coming directly from the plant) and add 1 desk spoon of honey.

Combine good all of the components, cover up your silver bowl with a lid and depart it to arrange for roughly 12 hours. Wipe your face with this renewing emulsion within the morning and, should you like, in the night, utilizing a cotton pad (you'll need to rinse it with water);

apply it for your face and neck and, when close to dry, reapply this cure again, do it for approximately 5-10 minutes; or make a facial compress for approx 5 minutes utilizing washcloth and this emulsion; then, rinse with heat water.

That you may maintain this emulsion within the fridge for about a week. This liquid mask can with ease breath youthfulness into your skin , renewing and nourishing it.

9-White clay masks once per week.

Cleopatra cherished traditional clays and knew methods to use them for magnificence. Right here is a simple face masks that the Egyptian Queen cherished: mix 2 table spoons of cosmetic white clay with three-four desk spoons of pure thermal water until you receive the paste. Follow this masks in your face for 5-10 minutes, however don't let it dry completely, because drying result may also be harsh on the skin.

Then, rinse this masks off your face with warm water. White clay has antiseptic residences and is rich in minerals and micro elements with a purpose to aid tone, carry, cleanse and renew your skin . Don't make this mask extra ordinarily than once per week.

10-Cleopatra adored to make use of rose water as a facial toner.

Luckily, we can now buy rose water in virtually any well being meals retailer or we can also prepare it ourselves. Wipe your face with rose water every morning and every night; use it, as a average face toner.

Rose water will surely make your skin   tender and soft, naturally hydrating and nourishing it.

That you would be able to additionally spray rose water to your face throughout the scorching summer day, it'll aid refresh and hydrate your skin , keeping it tender and supple. Rose water can be utilized on the face as an alternative of makeup primer – your groundwork will glide for your skin very easily and without problems; exclusive odor is a great bonus!

.

I am hoping you located these magnificence secrets and techniques of Cleopatra priceless.

Stay wonderful!

Disclaimer

The information contained on this book is intended for educational purposes only and is not a substitute for advice, diagnosis or treatment by a licensed physician.

It is not meant to cover all possible precautions, drug interactions, circumstances or adverse effects.

You should seek prompt medical care for any health issues and consult your doctor before using alternative medicine or making a change to your regime

About The Author

Biography

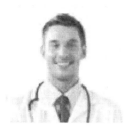

Dr. M. kotb is a board certified internist

Dr. Kotb is also medical director of the ELITE medical Center for internal medicine and Nutrition Studies,

which promotes

optimal nutrition through science-based education, advocacy,

and research in partnership with Hanover University, Germany

As medical director and chief medical editor at the training program of physicians, He now oversees a team of staff physicians and medical reviewers UK.

Responsible for creating content and assuring its continued medical accuracy and relevance

Dr. Kotb is a regular expert on national and local broadcast media, including regular appearances on UK Channels

He has also been interviewed by local and nationally syndicated radio stations, magazines, and newspapers across the country, speaking on everything from hangover remedies to navigating the Internet for accurate, credible health information.

Dr. Kotb serves as a member of the Nutrition Wellness Educator Certification Panel, established by the U.K. Association of Family Services.

The panel is responsible for determining the competency scope of the Nutrition Educator certification.

Dr. Kotb also volunteers at the Good medicine Health Center in Berkshire, where he sees patients who do not have health insurance or are unable to pay for health care.

As a board-certified internist, Dr. Kotb's interest and knowledge span a wide array of medical topics.

He is particularly interested in prevention and helping people live a healthy, active lifestyle

Dr. Kotb is a member of the international association of liver disease

He is A pioneer and internationally recognized expert in the fields of INTERVENTIONAL HEPATOLOGY,

DR M KOTB, MD is the creator of Be EXCELLENT, a proprietary brand of health coaching BOOKS.

He is A U.K. bestselling author WITH MORE than 200 books

He had been invited for over 150 oral presentations in conferences focusing primarily on family medicine

He is the Vice president of Berkshire charity for orphans.

For Correspondence:

London

Name: Mohamed Elkotb

Address Line1: Old Bath Road Colnbrook

Address Line2: JED 769904

City: Slough

State: Berkshire

ZipCode: SL3 0NS

Tel: 01753-210399

Learn more about DR KOTB at amazon.com/author page

You can discover my facebook fanpage here ➜

https://www.facebook.com/Neverseenbefore.co.uk/

you can join my email list here ➜

https://app.getresponse.com/site2/irresistibles?u=SuFzh&webforms_id=ALRG

Other Books by DR KOTB

How To Stop Binge Eating In Easy Steps : The Amazing Scientific Program To Heal Your Body , Stop Overeating , and get a supermodel fitness shape (Stop Binge Eating- Stop Overeating Book 1)

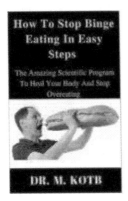

http://amzn.to/2CKnUIc

TRIPLE YOUR ORGASM : The amazing New Scientific program that will enhance male climax by beating the three monsters: erectile dysfunction, Premature Ejaculation ... health And Please your beloved Book 1)

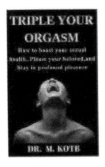

http://amzn.to/2FdW6gJ

THE FIBROMYALGIA-REVERSAL PROGRAM (MADE EASY) :The New Scientifically Proven Therapy To fix Fibromyalgia pain And reverse Chronic Fatigue In 6 Weeks

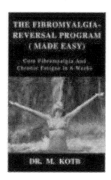

http://amzn.to/2CI00Nt

HOW TO BEAT THE KRYPTONITE The proven 12 steps protocol from the top successful ADHD superwomen to sister, wife, mother with Attention Deficit Disorder

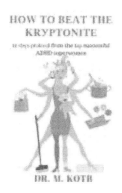

http://amzn.to/2DcLNZC

Add VA-VA-VOOM To Your Bedroom:The Advanced Art Of Beating Erectile Dysfunction AND The Step By Step Program For Profound Pleasuring Your Partner

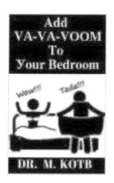

http://amzn.to/2m94MMG

MOOD CURE BY SCHEHERAZADE THERAPY : The new scientific program of Mood Therapy to Overcome Depression (Fast Depression Cure Book 1)

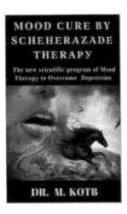

http://amzn.to/2CTlhaV

The SUMO Strategy to Reverse Diabetes-(The METABOLISM RESET AND INSULIN RESISTANCE SOLUTION)-The Amazing STEP by STEP Program To Reverse Diabetes And Pre-Diabetes ... In 7 Weeks

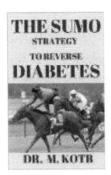

http://amzn.to/2mbPjeW

Fix your Weak Bladder : Must know things before buying bladder INCONTINENCE control products - How to choose the best product that works for you to Improve ... and overactive Bladder Control Book 1)

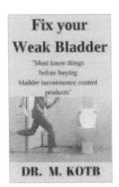

http://amzn.to/2ClioWk

The ADHD DIET : A STEP-BY-STEP GUIDE TO HOPE AND HEALING Attention Deficit Disorder BY LIVING GLUTEN FREE AND CASEIN FREE (GFCF) AND OTHER INTERVENTIONS (AUTISM and the ADHD DIET

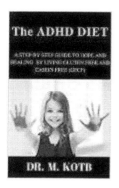

http://amzn.to/2mbPuXE

Think like your colon :How to cure your diverticulitis in amazing easy 3 steps-the scientific proven Diet guide for People with Diverticulitis and diverticulosis-plus ... diverticulitis and diverticulosis

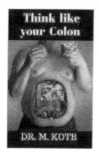

http://amzn.to/2AlY9pv

Pamper your liver: how to reset your fatty liver metabolism-The proven step by steps health program to reverse your insulin resistance and cure your fatty liver (all Natural,no Meds,no Budget,no Gym)

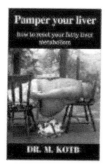

Killing 3 birds with one stone : The Scientifically Proven program to Reverse Heart Disease ,
Lower Blood Pressure and Lower cholesterol in 21 days

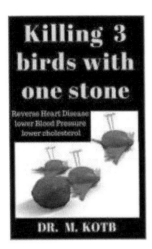

STILL SEXY UNDER FIRE : How To Have A FASCINATING Sex Life And Keep Romance Alive EVEN IF
You Have Multiple Sclerosis M.S.

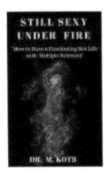

Brain Rules For Panic Sons : A 99 Proven Ways To Relief Panic Attacks, Harmonize Your Brain
Anxiety And Rebuild Your Relationships At Home And Work

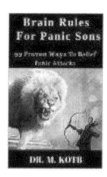

http://amzn.to/2DaoVtW

The Leaky gut miracle:The proven 7 steps program for Healing leaky gut and ibs by the healthy low FODMAP diet and Probiotics to skyrocket your wellness ... system (Healing leaky gut and IBS

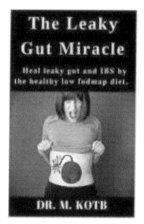

http://amzn.to/2CVuJe7

Candida Cure Diet : The proven Step by Step vibrant health Plan for recurring Candida Yeast, Fungus To Cleanse and reset Your immune System , Restore a ... (breakthrough candida-cure program

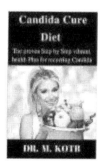

http://amzn.to/2CVPcyE

IMMUNOMANIA:The 100 Worst Mistakes You Are Doing In Your Autoimmune Solution Protocol-The Trusted Expert Guide To Avoid Health Mistakes Of Your Immune Reset Program,Prevent And Reverse Inflammation

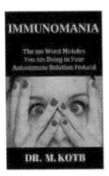

http://amzn.to/2CVPmGg

The Regretful butterfly: 100 Worst Mistakes you may make in your hypothyroidism solution protocol-The Trusted Expert Guide To Avoid Mistakes In Treating

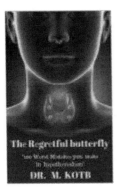

http://amzn.to/2CSSyCb

I tried the Limitless Pill of the silicon valley: The Must Know 100 Mistakes When Choosing Nootropics, Smart Drugs And Brain Enhancing Supplements

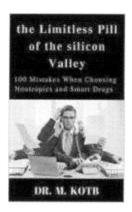

http://amzn.to/2CHAYhr

The 7 days ALCOHOL EXORCISM PROGRAM : The Amazing step by step Program To Get Rid Of Alcohol Addiction And Achieve Sobriety In 7 Days

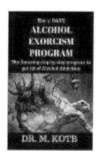

http://amzn.to/2D92ZiK

The Regretful pancreas : 100 Worst Mistakes you may make in your diabetes reversal protocol- The trusted expert guide to avoid mistakes in reversing your ... fatigue and get a Healthy pregnancy)

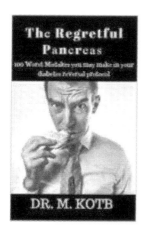

http://amzn.to/2CQupwh

Beat the thief of mind : The ultimate Caregiver's Guide to the most challenging situations in caring for People with Alzheimer and Dementia: Bowel and ... People with Alzheimer and Dementia

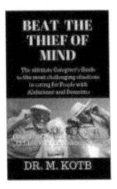

http://amzn.to/2CJ71xj

The supplement ultimate guide of the pros : How to use The proven science of supplements to Maximize Your Muscle and loose fat through workouts, weight ... ,Tribulus Terrestris , BCAA, ZMA and CLA)

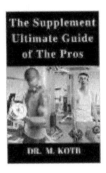

http://amzn.to/2m985U6

THE MICROBIOME CLIMAX : THE REVOLUTIONARY STEP BY STEP PROVEN GUIDE FOR USING GUT MICROBIOME – SEX CONNECTION TO IMPROVE LIBIDO IN WOMEN (BY 400 % IN 10 DAYS)

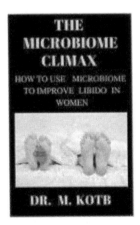

The Guaranteed Sleep Miracle :The Scientific Proven Step by Step Strategy to Harmonize Your Sleep,Your Body And Sex -Must Know Secrets of Diet, Neurofeedback ... Asleep FAST

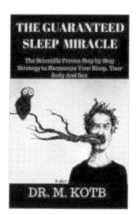

100 Amazing Secrets to a Perfect Memory : A step by step FUN and NATURAL program to improve and BOOST your Memory Power (HOW TO MAKE THE PILL THAT ERASES BAD MEMORIES)

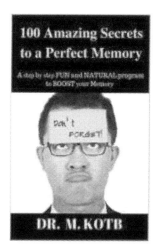

One Last Thing...

If you enjoyed this book or found it useful I'd be very grateful if you'd post a short review on Amazon.

Your support really does make a difference and I read all the reviews personally so I can get your feedback and make this book even better.

Thanks again for your support!

Printed in Great Britain
by Amazon